Grower's Reference on Gamebird Health

L. Dwight Schwartz

Correspondence regarding this *Grower's Reference on Gamebird Health* should be addressed to:

AVICON, Inc.,
3871 Sandlewood Drive,
Okemos, MI
48864

ISBN 0-9644732-0-8 29.95

Distributed by AVICON, Inc., Okemos, MI, USA

ABOUT OUR COVER:
  Original art: JAMES A. RENDER, DVM, PhD, Diplomate ACVP
  Detailed art: MARGARET (MAGGIE) R. HOFMANN

GROWERS' REFERENCE

ON

GAMEBIRD HEALTH

(CONTINUES)

(CONTINUED)

(CONTINUES)

(CONTINUED)

(CONTINUES)

(CONCLUDED)

FOREWORD

I have known Dr. Dwight Schwartz for more years than I care to mention. Dr. Schwartz has worked in the field of Avian Pathology since 1959. I must have first met him in the 1960s when Penn State University started holding its first gamebird conferences.

Dwight's appointments have led to faculty positions at three major universities (Georgia, Penn State, and Michigan State). He retired, Professor Emeritus, from the College of Veterinary Medicine at Michigan State in 1993. That seemed to be the only way he could manage time to compile and edit this much-needed book.

Dr. Schwartz is the author of four editions of *The Penn State Poultry Health Handbook*. That excellent manual was first published in 1972, and most recently revised in 1994. We have used a tremendous amount of information compiled by Dr. Schwartz.

His interests have always been with gamebirds. Dwight has been an advisor and 'guiding light' to the gamebird industry. He has made educational presentations at innumerable gamebird conferences. He has written numerous articles on gamebird diseases for *WILDLIFE HARVEST* and other publications.

This *Grower's Reference on Gamebird Health* is the first reference written specifically for the gamebird producer in the past 50 years. It addresses all aspects of commonly encountered gamebird diseases. It also addresses the 'rarely seen maladies' that may be found within certain regions of the nation.

I am proud to have had a hand in encouraging Dwight to write a book specifically on GAMEBIRD diseases. This book exceeds my expectations. Each disease coverage provides a concise, comprehensive overview of the malady (as well as the recommended treatment, control, and prevention).

The wealth of scientific information is presented in an easy-to-use format. It is written in a language that is understandable to the producer. As editor of Wildlife Harvest publications, I appreciate, admire, and encourage writing that is clear and easily understood.

JOHN M MULLIN
Clinton, IA
May 1, 1995

Editor's Note: John M Mullen is Information Officer, North American Gamebird Association and Editor & Publisher, WILDLIFE HARVEST Publications.

PREFACE

Gamebirds represent some of the most colorful and attractive birds in the world. Several species are raised for their economic importance as birds for sport hunting or as gourmet-food items. Millions of gamebirds are harvested annually by hunters in the wild and on regulated hunting preserves. Privately owned farms produce and supply gamebirds for the hunting and gourmet markets. Some of these birds are used to repopulate or establish gamebird populations in habitats.

Exotic and rare species of gamebirds are collected, bred, and maintained by hobbyists. Hobbyists are attracted to gamebirds for their beauty. Collections normally include rare and exotic breeds as well as the more common breeds. Many aspects of husbandry for domestic and exotic breeds are similar yet differ in pairing, mating, and the amount of space required for the breeding stock, housing, nutrition, egg care, and incubation.

This book was written primarily to help growers and others in the industry identify, understand, treat, control, and prevent infectious diseases that specifically affect gamebirds. Each disease or malady is addressed individually where it fits into the appropriate chapter for each etiological type. Chapters are divided into bacterial, viral, protozoan, parasitic, nutritional, metabolic, toxic, and miscellaneous conditions. Each disease is written in such a way to attempt to divide traits or specifics of causative-agent that are important to cure, eradicate, or establish control for the respective disorder. Disease treatment is more than prescribing medication. Husbandry, environmental, nutritional, etc., adjustments must be made as necessary for medicinal therapy to work.

Drugs and antibiotics are mentioned by name solely for the convenience of the producer in identifying the type of medication needed in treating a respective infection. The mention of a trade name is not to be interpreted, however, as an endorsement of that product alone. Likewise, failure to name a specific product does not imply a lack of endorsement. All drugs and antibiotics must be cleared by US Food and Drug Administration (FDA) for use in gamebirds, poultry, and animals. The gamebird producer is advised to use only products that have FDA clearance for their birds. Use of an "Extra-label" drug is safe only when prescribed by a licensed veterinarian; therefore, the veterinarian should be consulted for advice on specific medications and health problems.

L.D.S.
May 1, 1995

IN APPRECIATION —

It has been a labor of love for me to write the *Grower's Reference on Gamebird Health*. For many years, it has been my goal to create this book. I have known and worked with gamebird producers since 1960 so I readily recognize the need for a reliable book on diseases affecting gamebirds. The *Grower's Reference* has been written, in the spirit of service to the gamebird industry, to fulfill that need. I have drawn on a variety of scientific publications in assembling the text as no publication is developed without a bibliography of accurate current scientific resources. This book is no exception.

No publication is done without the help of many other reliable persons. Without their help, this book could not have been written or published. In addition, without the electronic marvel of the computer, this book would never have been considered. Those who worked so diligently to make this book a reality are:

EDITOR: My editor is Glenn D. Bengtson, founder and senior editor of After Sum Tymne Editors and Publishers, a very specialized house in State College, PA. I've worked with Bing for many years on a number of projects, including the first, third, and fouth editions of *The Penn State Poultry Health Handbook*. It was, I think, during our working up of the *Handbook's* Third Edition that we started to talk seriously about working together on a book for gamebird growers just as soon as we retired from our respective universities. But then Penn State requested a revision of the Third Edition and this gamebird book got laid aside for more than a few weeks.

Specifically, Bing edited the text, prepared the final paging, and provided advice on the book's general organization. His office made the arrangements with the printer and guided the book through manufacturing. He'll be quick to point out that Miriam (i.e., Mrs. Bengtson) played a key role in recording traffic, proofing, and, from time to time prodding. Wives are like that. That's why they're essential in all respects.

Mr. Bengtson is an agricultural journalist and editor who worked in this capacity for Pennsylvania State University until his retirement. His tenure at Penn State lead to assignments with international agricultural research centers in India and Africa. His work is recognized and appreciated world wide.

COVER: The cover was designed and drawn by Dr. James A Render, DVM, PHD, Diplomate ACVP. Dr. Render is a veterinary pathologist at the Animal Health Diagnostic Laboratory, College of Veterinary

Medicine, Michigan State University. Dr. Render has a gifted artistic talent he is using in several ways, including the design of covers for scientific publications.

COVER DEVELOPMENT: Margaret R. (Maggie) Hofmann, staff graphic artist for the College of Veterinary Medicine, Michigan State University. Maggie used her graphic arts skills to develop the style, cover layout, balance of bird profile, and prepare the camera-ready art from the cover created by Dr. Render.

TEXT DESIGN: Last but certainly not least is Wilma J. Schwartz, my wife, who deciphered the text from my hand-written manuscript. She was responsible for text design, page format, word processing, sentence structure, punctuation, and preliminary editing. Wilma had an integral role in the writing of *Grower's Reference on Gamebird Health*. Without her assistance, the book could not have been published.

Of course, I also must acknowledge the assistance and encouragement of the vast number of colleagues, Association members, growers, teachers, and friends that over the years have provided assistance, encouragement, and insight. This book reflects the combined effort of all, and I am grateful for it.

L.D.S.
May 1, 1995

GROWER'S REFERENCE

ON

GAMEBIRD HEALTH

BY

L. DWIGHT SCHWARTZ, D.V.M., M.S.

— LISTING OF SECTIONS —

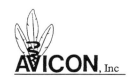

AVICON, Inc

CODES AND MEASUREMENTS

SC: Subcutaneous injection (under the skin)

WD: Withdrawal time (days required for drugs to clear tissues)

IM: Intramuscular injection (into the muscle)

C: Continuous use

d/w: day/week and days/weeks

g: gram

gal: gallon

kg: kilogram (1000 g)

ltr: liter

mg: milligram

ml: milliliter

oz: ounce

pk: packet

ppm: parts per million

pt: pint

qt: quart

tsp: teaspoon

tbs: tablespoon

T: ton (2 000 lb)

LIQUID MEASURES WITH METRIC EQUIVALENTS:

1 tsp = 1/3 tbs = 5 ml

3 tsp = 1 tbs = 1/2 oz = 15 ml (approx.)

6 tsp = 2 tbs = 1 oz = 30 ml (approx.)

1 cup = 1/2 pt = 8 oz = 250 ml (approx.)

1 pt = 2 cups = 16 oz = 500 ml (approx.)

1 qt = 2 pt = 32 oz = 1000 ml (approx)

1 gal = 4 qt = 128 oz = 3.8 ltr

DRY MEASURES WITH METRIC EQUIVALENTS

1 oz = 29 g

1 lb = 16 oz = 454 g

1 kg = 2.2 lb = 1000 g

1 g = 1000 mg

1 ppm = 1 g/T = 1 mg/kg

GROWERS' REFERENCE

ON

GAMEBIRD HEALTH

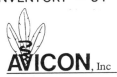

AVICON, Inc

LENGTH OF INCUBATION PERIODS OF PATHOGENS
and
COURSES OF IMPORTANT INFECTIOUS DISEASES

H = hour or hours   D = day or days
W = week or weeks   M = month or months
depop'n = depopulation

PATHOGENS or DISEASES	INCUBATION	COURSE
Aspergillosis	4 to 10 D	Acute: 2 to 6 W
		Chronic: 1 to 3 M
Avian Encephalomyelitis (AE)	10 to 17 D	2 to 4 W
Avian Influenza (AI)	3 to 5 D	10 to 28 D
Avian Tuberculosis (TB)	W to M	Chronic
Avian Pox	4 to 10 D	Slow /W
Bordetella avium	7 to 9 D	2 to 6 W
Botulism	H (lethal)	4 to 24 H
Campylobacter Hepatitis	5 to 15 D	3 W - long
Candidiasis	7 to 21 D	Chronic
Chlamydiosis	5 to 7 D	Slow to long
Colibacillosis	2 to 3 D	2 to 6 W
Derzsy's Disease	4 to 7 D	3 to 5 W
Duck Virus Enteritis (DVE)	3 to 7 D	3 to 4 D
Duck Virus Hepatitis (DVH)	1 to 2 D	3 to 4 D
Equine Encephalitis (EE)	2 to 5 D	2 to 4 W
Erysipelas	2 to 3 D	2 to 4 W
Fowl Cholera (FC)	3 to 9 D	2 W/depop'n
Fowl Typhoid	4 to 5 D	3 to 5 W
Goose Septicemia (Past.)	3 to 9 D	2 W/depop'n
Inclusion Body Hepatitis (IBH)	1 to 3 D	10 to 13 D
Infectious Coryza (Hemophilus)	1 to 3 D	4 to 12 W
Laryngotracheitis (LT)	2 to 12 D	7 to 14 D
Listeriosis	36 H to 52 D	1 to 14 D
Marble Spleen Disease (MSD)	6 to 8 D	1 to 3 W
Mycoplasma Gallisepticum (MG)	3 to 10 D	Slow/long
Mycoplasma Meleagridis (MM)	5 to 10 D	Slow/long
Mycoplasma Synoviae (MS) Turkeys	5 to 10 D	Slow/long
Necrotic Enteritis (NE)	3 to 6 D	10 to 14 D
Newcastle Disease (ND)	5 to 7 D	10 to 14 D

(CONTINUES)

INCUBATION TIMES AND COURSE PERIODS (CONCLUDED)

H = hour or hours   D = day or days
W = week or weeks   M = month or months
Depop'n = depopulation

PATHOGEN DISEASES	INCUBATION	COURSE
Omphalitis (Navel Ill)	H	6 to 7 D
Paratyphoid	4 to 5 D	3 to 5 W
Pasteurella (Riemerella) anatipestifer	3 to 9 D	3 to 5 W
Pigeon Paramyxovirus-I (PMV-1)	2 to 7 D	10 to 14 D
Pullorum Disease	4 to 5 D	3 to 5 W
Quail Bronchitis (QB)	4 to 7 D	3 to 5 W
Rotavirus Enteritis	2 to 5 D	3 to 4 W
Spirochetosis	3 to 5 D	3 to 5 W
Staphylococcosis	1 to 3 D	3 to 5 W
Streptococcosis	1 to 3 D	5 to 21 D
Transmissible Enteritis (TE)	2 to 3 D	10 to 14 D
Ulcerative Enteritis(Quail Disease)	3 to 6 D	2 to 6 W

HEALTH MAINTENANCE

INTRODUCTION AND FUNDAMENTALS

Outbreaks of infectious diseases in gamebirds and poultry normally originate from one or more of the following methods:

INFECTED BIRDS BROUGHT ON TO THE FARM: New birds include newly hatched birds, started or immature birds, and adult birds for breeders or other uses.

RECOVERED CARRIER BIRDS: Birds kept from the previous year's production that have recovered from an endemic disease on the premises. In other words, recovered birds remain carriers and shedders of the disease.

INADEQUATE CLEANING AND DISINFECTION (C& D) AND BASIC SANITATION: Short cuts in building and/or pen decontamination permits the causative organisms to remain within the pen or facility. During pre-season preparation is the opportune time to thoroughly decontaminate pen facilities and equipment, thus assuring a disease-free production season.

FAULTY BIOSECURITY: Biosecurity is doing those things necssary to absolutely prevent the introduction of infectious contagious diseases by the normal entry channels. Biosecurity includes: keeping out unauthorized persons, locking doors, insect control, and routine sanitary measures.

VECTOR CONTROL: This is directed toward the control of particular insects, such as mosquitoes, black flies, biting midges, and other specific insects that are known to spread certain disease(s). Mosquitoes spread Avian pox and equine encephalitis (EE), black flies and biting midges spread malarial-type diseases.

RODENT CONTROL: Rodent feces have been found to contain high numbers of Salmonella and other potentially infectious bacteria. Besides spreading disease to gamebird pens, rodents carry the same diseases to nearby houses and outdoor bird pens. Rodent control must be vigorous and ongoing.

Rodents are strongly attracted to bird-rearing facilities because of the ready feed supply and shelter. Actual rodent numbers are many times higher than those seen by the caretaker. The grower should become familiar with feeding and breeding habits of various rodents, especially mice and rats. Control measures for mice and rats are: (i) elimi-nate nesting-hiding materials and places inside and outside the buildings; (ii) seal entry holes; (iii) repair broken concrete; (iv) rodent-proof feed bins and/or feed-storage rooms; (v) establish bait stations and set traps. Baiting and traps work very well just after a building has been depopulated.

Good poultry house sanitation begins with a clean, disinfected house, prepared well (at least 2 weeks) before placement of new birds. The effectiveness of sanitization of a facility depends on the thoroughness of cleaning and washing before a germicide is applied. Thorough C& D is essential because it reduces pathogen load, removes materials that provide refuge to pathogens, and exposes surfaces to light, air, and disinfectants.

FUNDAMENTALS OF HEALTH MAINTENANCE

1.   Preventive medicine is the only logical approach to health man-agement in today's intensive gamebird operations. As flock size dou-bles, the possibilities of disease quadruple.

2.   Preventive medicine includes disease-free hatchlings, good hus-bandry, medication, and adequate nutrition — performed under good sanitation and biosecurity.

3.   Thoroughly clean and disinfect (C&D) house and equipment af-ter each group of birds. Put in new litter. Compost used litter to de-stroy source of disease carry-over.

4.   Pullorum-test breeders or buy from NPIP-member producers.

5.   Keep young birds well isolated from older birds. Separate facili-ties and caretakers will increase chances of successful isolation.

6.   Isolate poultry from other livestock. Chickens, cattle, gamebirds, turkeys, and swine are subject to cross-infections.

7.   Provide nutritionally balanced feed, commercial or home-mixed.

8.   Provide a continuous supply of potable water for all birds. In summer, keep the water cool by providing shade; in winter, protect from freezing. Birds consume up to 2.5 times as much water as feed. When water-intake decreases, there is a proportionate decrease in feed intake. Marked reductions in feed and water consumption are usually the first signs of illness.

9.   Do not crowd birds. Crowding increases cannibalism, feather

picking, hysteria, and other stress-related problems. Crowding retards growth, reduces feed efficiency, and decreases production.

10. During brooding, regulate temperature, humidity, and ventilation to the comfort of the brooding birds. Prevent drafts, overheating, and chilling.

11. Keep unauthorized and unnecessary personnel out of the gamebird facility. Discourage unnecessary visits to your facilities and to other poultry operations.

12. Incineration is the safest, in terms of health of surviving birds, method of dead bird disposal. Composting or deep burying, in that order, are the next best methods. Dead birds, if not disposed of, become a disease threat to other gamebirds and poultry in the area.

13. In disease outbreaks, promptly obtain a reliable diagnosis. Then use the best treatment for that specific disease. Birds recovered from diseases like pullorum and mycoplasmosis are reservoirs of disease, and should not be saved for breeder replacements.

14. It is best that you accompany your diseased or dead birds to the diagnostic laboratory; in this way you will be available to provide additional information that might be needed.

BIOSECURITY

Biosecurity is safety or protection from transmission of infectious agents of any type — viral, bacterial, fungal, or parasitic. Emergency and common diseases are produced by microbes or germs that are invisible except when viewed under a modern microscope. In less than a day, a single microbe can produce and multiply to a number greater than the number of people on earth. Microbes are our enemy. They are killers. Keeping these disease agents off your premises and out of your gamebirds is the key to flock health and success of your business. BIOSECURITY KEEPS GAMEBIRDS FREE FROM DISEASE!

HOW TO ENFORCE BIOSECURITY? Keep buildings and premises locked. Always change to fresh, clean coveralls, hat, and boots when visiting a farm or moving from one farm to another. People are the biggest threat to biosecurity. Equipment used on farms should be cleaned, washed, and disinfected before it is moved to another farm. If possible, have separate equipment for each farm. Pay careful attention to hauling crates, egg cases, delivery trucks, feeders, and waterers, and to loaders and dumpsters, tractors, tool boxes, pickup trucks, vaccine sprayers, and debeakers.

WHAT ARE OTHER PREVENTIVE MEASURES? Plan and engineer your operations to prevent situations that may expose your flock to disease. Schedule equipment and house repairs for after your flock has been marketed. Provide a simple room where visitors may change clothes. Invest in a supply of smooth-soled rubber or strong-soled plastic boots for visitors' use.

Good ventilation pays! Large amounts of fresh air dilute microbe populations and reduce disease buildup. Place new poultry buildings and facilities as far as possible from other poultry operations and poultry traffic. Do business only with firms whose service people practice high biosecurity standards.

Biosecurity Dos and Do Nots

DOs:	DO NOTs:
Keep poultry comfortable.	Permit dirty coops, crates, etc., on your farm.
"All in-all out" management.	
C&D housing and equipment at least once a year.	Keep various types of fowl, including pet birds.
Compost, bury, or burn dead gamebirds.	House birds of different ages in one facility.
Prevent contact with songbirds, waterfowl, and seabirds.	Visit poultry on other farms.

USING THE POULTRY DIAGNOSTIC LABORATORY

Every gamebird producer is encouraged to become acquainted with the poultry diagnostic laboratory. The use of this facility to identify diseases, if accompanied by timely treatment can save the producer costly production losses. Any type of health or production problem can be submitted to the diagnostic laboratory. A laboratory diagnosis provides the producer with an accurate cause of the problem. Most pathologists at the laboratory can recommend or prescribe specific medication for the disease diagnosed. Specific medication normally provides a dramatic treatment response by comparison to no or little response to a wrong medication. Symptomatic therapy often leads to the use of the wrong medication in which the disease remains unchecked and bird mortality continues. Incorrect diagnosis and treatment adds to the cost of the problem. Producers should establish liveability standards for each gamebird species grown. When mortality is high, a laboratory diagnosis should be obtained. The problem must be identified in order to protect succeeding hatches.

POINTS REGARDING THE USE OF THE
POULTRY DIAGNOSTIC LABORATORY:

1. Accuracy of any diagnosis depends upon the information available to the diagnostician. This information, for the most part, comes from two sources — the birds submitted for necropsy and the facts supplied by the flock manager. Early identification of the disease and its cause will reduce treatment time and expense, and shorten the course of the disease, thereby reducing losses from mortality and reduced performance.

2. Always submit a few live birds for diagnosis, as the disease agent is more easily isolated from a freshly killed bird than from a bird that has been dead for several hours. A few freshly dead birds can be submitted. Decomposed birds are of no diagnostic value.

3. Select birds that most nearly represent the primary condition affecting the flock, not cull birds.

4. Try to select birds showing different stages of the disease. Viral and bacterial isolations are more easily accomplished when the disease is in its early stages, but the diagnostician may need to see advanced stages of the problem as well.

5. The number of birds in a useful specimen is somewhat depen-

dent on the age of the birds. Select six to eight birds in flocks less than 3 weeks old, five in flocks 3 to 12 weeks of age, four birds in flocks in 12 to 16 weeks of age, or three birds if older than 16 weeks.

6.   Be prepared to submit a second set of birds, in the event the diagnostician is unable to confirm identity of the disease with the initial submission.

TRANSPORTATION OF SPECIMENS:

1.   Transport live specimens in well-ventilated containers of sufficient size to avoid crowding, cramping, and suffocation of the birds.

2.   Containers must be burnable. Cardboard boxes are excellent and inexpensive.

3.   A detailed and complete history should accompany the birds. Even better, deliver your birds to the laboratory and talk with the diagnostician yourself. Watch the necropsy of your birds.

4.   Birds and containers should not be returned to the farm. THIS IS FUNDAMENTAL TO BIOSECURITY.

5.   If birds must be expressed or mailed, they should be sent by the fastest method. Pack dead birds in dry ice to avoid decomposition. Enclose the history, or attach it to the shipping container. Make sure the shipment is identified with your name, address, phone number, and fax number, and address, as well as the name, address, and phone and fax numbers of your veterinarian

MONITORING FLOCK HEALTH

Flock health monitoring is the procedure used to evaluate the health status of a flock at any given time. It is recommended that growers become familiar with necropsy techniques so they can routinely (on a weekly schedule) necropsy and examine all birds that die on a given day of the week. In cases of sudden increase in bird mortality, all dead birds should be examined to determine the types of lesions present. Record and tally lesions found daily on dead birds. Also record other peculiar signs of illness noted on a day-to-day basis. This information is extremely valuable when submitting birds to a pathology laboratory or veterinarian for diagnosis.

Most good gamebird managers become adept at necropsy as a means to monitor the current diseases that threaten their flocks. Learn how to recognize and describe the lesions found in your dead birds. The following procedural outline will be helpful for you to train yourself in the examination and necropsy of dead birds.

Birds that have been dead for a period of time are of limited value for necropsy purposes. A live bird that is representative of the malady is preferable. For laboratory submission, include several freshly dead as well as sick live birds.

1.   Carefully consider the flock history, i.e., clinical signs, species, breed, age, vaccination, feed, drug treatment, and other pertinent information.

2.   Observe the general appearance and condition of the birds for symptoms and external lesions (eye, skin, feathers, fleshing, lice or mites, etc.).

3.   Blood specimen, plate tests, blood smears and hematocrits must be done before birds are killed (if indicated for diagnosis).

4.   Method of killing:

ADULT BIRDS: Use cervical disarticulation by placing the thumb of the right hand on the base of the skull. Grasp the legs of the bird in the left hand and pull. Rotate the right hand slightly and the neck joint will be disarticulated.

CHICKS, SMALL, OR BABY BIRDS: Use handle of scissors over the neck to crush or rupture the neck and spinal cord.

5.   Again check the bird for external lesions. Do not pull feathers from the bird. Loose feathers create a messy room that is difficult to

clean.

6. Place the dead or freshly killed bird on its back on the work table with its head away from the operator. Feathers may be dampened, if desired, to minimize feather dust.

7. Incise the skin between each thigh and disarticulate each leg at hip joint. Incise the skin posterior to the keel and reflect the skin forward, exposing all the breast muscle and the ventral surface of the neck. Next, reflect the skin over the legs to expose front border of thigh muscles for signs of hemorrahage on fat and fascia. Examine the breast and leg muscles for hemorrhage, bruises and other abnormalities.

8. Cut the femur (mid-shaft) with shears to examine bone marrow (fat in marrow is anemia).

9. Examine the leg bones by removing the muscle tissue. Test the tensile strength of bones, especially in baby chicks, by breaking the tibia (there should be a sharp snap when the bone breaks). Examine the joints for infection. The hock joint is most frequently affected.

10. Transversely incise the abdominal muscles posterior to the keel. Insert the point of necropsy shears into the abdominal cavity and cut forward through the abdominal muscles and costochondral junction of the ribs on a horizontal plane. Extend the cut through the shoulder girdle on each side. Do not cut into the lungs.

11. Examine the pericardial sac and air sacs (cervical and clavicular) and inner surface of the keel as you lift the sternum away from the bird.

12. The ventral surfaces of the viscera are now exposed, allowing you to examine the internal organs in their normal position.

13. Grasp the liver and gizzard and move them from side to side gently to allow examination of the thoracic abdominal air sacs.

14. Pick up the proventriculus and sever the esophagus just anterior to the proventriculus. Displace the proventriculus, gizzard, and entire intestinal tract posteriorly. Do not destroy the loop of the duodenum to allow you to later examine the pancreas. Examine outer surface of the intestines. Open the entire intestinal tract and examine the contents for internal parasites and mucosal lining for enteritis and hemorrhage. Do not put water in the abdominal cavity.

15. Remove liver and spleen. They may be rinsed in running tap

water. Examine each thoroughly.

16. Observe the heart in position, then remove and examine it.

17. Examine the ovaries, oviduct or testicles.

18. Examine the kidneys in position.

19. Examine the lungs in position. Next, break loose the air sacs and serous coverings of the lungs. Begin at the posterior lateral edge of the lungs to strip them out medially (toward center of carcass). Examine the external and cut surfaces of the lungs.

20. Take out the trachea and examine.

21. Examine the turbinates and sinuses by making a transverse cut between the nostrils and eyes.

22. Examine the esophagus and crop. Begin at one corner of the mouth with scissors to open the esophagus and crop. Examine the contents and lining.

23. Examine the brain — cut away skull cap carefully. Do not mutilate brain tissue.

24. Arrange for laboratory tests (cultures, virus isolations, histopathology) needed.

Often it will be necessary to examine organs for micro-organisms for histopathology; therefore, do not destroy or grossly contaminate organs until diagnostic cultures can be made and tissue specimens can be saved.

HUSBANDRY AND SANITATION

The practice of husbandry and sanitation means providing healthful, nurturing care for bird and animal rearing. Husbandry requires the ultimate in environmental preparation of the brooding/rearing facility. To remain disease-free, birds need adequate, clean, and sanitary feeding-drinking space, heat and ventilation, fresh nutritionally balanced feed (complete diet), and clean potable water. Understanding the rearing requirements of each type of bird is essential, because growth requirements and disease susceptibility vary with each gamebird species.

Husbandry is keeping the feeders-waterers clean and free of slime and seeing that the litter is fresh and dry. Waterers require frequent cleaning and sanitizing because of feed and fecal contamination. Contamination by feed or fecal matter introduces harmful bacteria into the water. Water at room temperature fosters rapid growth of bacteria, as may be noted by the water becoming cloudy and slime accumulating on the wall of the water trough. Husbandry also means keeping the birds comfortable and safe — effective biosecurity. Maintaining brooder and/or house temperatures at a comfortable level and providing ample feed and water for all birds at all times is a husbandry function.

WHAT IS SANITATION? Sanitation is the promotion of good health by using hygiene and cleanliness techniques that eliminate or reduce disease-causing organisms in the environment. Diseases are reduced and controlled in a sanitary environment. Hygiene must be a routine part of all gamebird-management programs.

Sanitation principles must be practiced by all people that visit gamebird farms. This includes service and equipment personnel.

If a contagious disease should occur, complete cleaning and decontamination must be achieved before repopulating the farm. In many cases, such as the California Newcastle epidemic, sentinel (susceptible) birds were used to determine if decontamination goals were met.

In addition to the poultry house, proper sanitation practices must be applied to egg handling, hatchery equipment, vehicles, and people. In this regard, each phase of a gamebird operation may require the use of different products and procedures.

CLEANING AND DISINFECTING (C&D)[1]

BIRD REMOVAL

A. Remove all dead and live birds from building; this includes all escaped (free-running) birds.

B. Immediately begin vector-control procedures for flies, beetles, mosquitos, and rodents.

DRY CLEANING

A. Clean fans and other air inlets from the outside.

B. On the inside, brush, sweep, vacuum, and wipe dust and other dirt from ceilings, light fixtures, beams, ledges, walls, fans, air inlets, and walkways. MOVE FROM TOP TO BOTTOM.

C. Promptly open feeder lines and remove feed from trough, all line corners, and all other points of feed accumulation.

D. Hard-surface (concrete) floors can be cleaned faster and more easily than clay or earthen floors. Completely remove all litter. Hand sweeping and shoveling will be necessary around the perimeter, doorways, walks, and support poles, and the corners of most houses to do a satisfactory job. If possible, fill manure trailers inside the houses and cover before moving to a disposal or composting site. Manure should not be spread near poultry facilities.

E. Turn off power to electrical equipment prior to dry or wet cleaning. Nonremovable motors, switches, etc., must be dry cleaned with compressed air or brushing. Extreme care should be taken to not get any water inside electric motors. Duct tape can be used to cover the slots in motor housings prior to wet cleaning and disinfection. The tape must be removed after wet cleaning and disinfection is completed.

WET CLEANING

Wet cleaning includes soaking, washing, and rinsing. Use of hot water is preferred. Detergents added to the washing solution will loosen debris and break down films to allow better penetration of cleaning agents.

Bacteria can multiply to high numbers in the presence of debris and moisture. Therefore, the following steps should be executed without interim waiting periods:

---

[1] Adapted with written permission from USAHA Subcommittee, Best Management Practices for Salmonella Risk Reduction in Broilers.

A. Soften dirt in heavily soiled areas. A low-pressure (200 to 300 psi) sprayer, delivering 10 to 30 gal/min is adequate.

B. Washing. Start at the back and work toward the front of the building, spraying the ceiling first, then the walls, and finally the floor. Use sprayer attachments and nozzles that permit washing hard-to-reach areas.

1. Wash ceiling and walls. Clean everything completely. Although use of pressure sprays ranging from 200-2000 psi has been reported, washing pressures of 750 to 2000 psi appear to be preferred. At high pressure, however, special care and safety garments are needed. Pressure sprayers can cut human skin like a knife. Care must be exercised to follow the manufacturer's instructions while using this equipment.

2. Pay special attention not only to the top, but also to the undersurfaces of troughs and hidden surfaces of chains and augers.

3. Wash storage rooms, hallways, break, wash-up, and restrooms.

4. Manually clean any areas that have resisted prior cleaning.

C. Rinsing.

1. To obtain a truly clean building, a final rinse to reduce residues of cleaning chemicals is suggested.

2. Immediately remove all puddles. Puddled water becomes a bacterial breeding ground.

REPAIRS

All repairs should be made at this point.

INSPECTION

Third-party visual inspection for completeness of the wet cleaning and repair operations is recommended.

DISINFECTING

Disinfecting should begin within 24 hours of rinsing. Do not begin until the house has passed its inspection for proper cleaning.

A. Heat Enhancement. All disinfectants, whether sprays, foams, aerosols, or fumigants, work best at temperatures above 65°F. Temperatures for chlorine- and iodine-based disinfectants should not exceed 110°F.

B. Dangerous Mixtures. Each disinfectant is the result of careful formulation, and the addition of detergents, surfactants, or insecticides to the disinfectant without the approval of its manufacturer could dangerously reduce its efficiency. Product label instructions must be followed carefully.

C. Evaluation of Products. Table 1 (p 19) provides guidance on evaluating efficacy of various products.

D. One gallon of diluted disinfectant is ordinarily applied to approximately 100-150 sq ft of surface area.

E. Follow application instructions of the manufacturer. Pressure spray is advisable to help force disinfectants into wood pores, cracks and crevices. Spray pressures of 500-1000 psi have been suggested. Move from back to front and from top to bottom.

F. Dirt floors are virtually impossible to fully disinfect. In situations where concrete has not been used to replace dirt floors, disinfectant has been applied to the floor at 1 gallon diluted disinfectant per 10 sq ft. Favorable results are reported with Clorox and formaldehyde. Note formaldehyde warning below.

G. Formaldehyde Fumigation Warning: FORMALDEHYDE AND FORMALIN ARE DANGEROUS CHEMICALS! Consequently, contact state/federal (EPA, OSHA, FDS) authorities and licensed professionals before considering use! Gas masks, protective clothing, and rescue plans are essential.

H. Promptly dry the building. Portable space heaters have been used to speed drying in cold and damp climates.

PREPARATION FOR RESTARTING

A. Remove old water filters. Clean and disinfect casing and install new filters.

B. Remove coverings and tape used to protect electrical circuits and motors and make sure that all electrical equipment, time clocks, feed and water lines, brooder stoves, etc. operate properly.

C. All decontamination equipment such as rakes, shovels, scrapers, brushes, trucks, manure spreaders, bucket loaders and spray/disinfection devices also should be cleaned and disinfected after use and stored in a secure location.

TABLE 1. PROPERTIES AND EXAMPLES OF COMMON DISINFECTANTS[1]

SPECIAL PROPRERTIES	HYPOCHLORIDES CHLORAMINES	IODOPHORS	CREOSOLS PHENOLS
Active against gram negative bacteria (*E. coli*, Salmonella, etc.)	Yes	Yes	Yes
Resistance to organic debris	Poor	Poor to fair	Good
Effects with hard water	None[2]	None	None
Heat detrimental	Yes	Yes	Yes
Residual activity	Yes	Yes	Yes
Most effective pH range	Acidic	Acidic	Acidic
Compatible with anionic surfactants (soaps)	Yes	Yes	Yes
Compatible with nonanionic surfactants	Yes	Yes	No

COMMON BRANDS AND NAMES

	HYPOCHLORIDES CHLORAMINES	IODOPHORS	CREOSOLS PHENOLS
	Chloramine-T	Betadine	Cresl-400
	Chlorox	Bio-Dyne	Environ-D
	Halazone	Iofec	LpH-AG
		Isodyne	Lysol
		Losan	Orthophenyl-phenols
		Tamed Iodine	Pd 2556
			Tek-Trol

[1] Modified from *Biosecurity for Poultry* (Brunet) and *Selection and Use of Disinfectants in Disease Prevention* (Meyerhols and Gaskin),

[2] Unless hard water is alkaline

DISINFECTANTS AND GERMICIDES

The information below is provided as a guide to selecting an effective disinfectant for your specific need. Frequently, identical or nearly identical compounds are marketed under different trade names and the concentration of active ingredients may vary. All products are required by law to be properly labeled with the chemical nature of the product and with instruction for its safe and effective use.

QUATERNARY AMMONIUM COMPOUNDS (QUATS): Quats are effective against a wide variety of microorganisms, including some fungi and viruses, but are not effective against bacterial or fungal spores. The compounds are fast-acting, odorless, nonirritating, noncorrosive, relatively nontoxic. The effectiveness of quats is reduced by soaps and detergents. Hard water also reduces their effectiveness.

COAL TAR DISTILLATES: Numerous disinfectants are based on cresylic acid and xylenols obtained from coal tar distillates. Coal tar distillates vary in effectiveness, but most are active against bacteria, some fungi, and some viruses. Coal tar distillates are fast-acting, have residual activity, and are not affected by hard water or organic matter.

IODINE COMPOUNDS: All are broad spectrum in their antibacterial action but only slightly effective against bacterial and fungal spores. Iodine compounds are fast-acting and effective against some viruses. Organic matter adversely affects their activity.

SYNTHETIC PHENOLS: Vary widely in effectiveness due to compositional differences. Synthetic phenols are effective against some bacteria, fungi, and some viruses but are not effective against bacterial spores. Phenols act rapidly and are resistant to inactivation by organic matter.

CHLORINE COMPOUNDS: Usually are hypochlorites that release active chlorine that is effective against most bacteria, fungi, some bacterial spores and some viruses. They are unaffected by hard water, kill very rapidly, have little residual activity.

FUMIGANTS: Formaldehyde, formalin, and paraformaldehyde are not commonly used in gamebird houses or on equipment. They are frequently used in hatcheries and incubators.

CAUTION: Select the appropiate disinfecting compound for the job at hand and follow instructions carefully. Errors can be costly in terms of time, money, and health of your birds.

KEYS TO SUCCESSFUL INCUBATION

The egg is nature's most perfectly self-contained life package. It holds a single fertilized egg cell, surrounded by nutrients so finely balanced that the cell needs only a congenial environment to grow into a chick. The basic environmental conditions of incubation are simple, but even minor deviations will bring down hatching percentages and may cause total loss of the hatch. Commercial hatching percentages usually exceed 75 percent.

CARE OF THE HATCHING EGG

Eggs for hatching should be stored at 55°F to 65°F and at a relative humidity of between 80 and 90 percent. Hatching percentages drop after eggs have been held for 7 days. If held beyond 7 days, eggs should be stored, large end up, at angles of 30 to 40 degrees from the vertical. The tilt should be reversed every day to prevent the yolk from sticking to the shell membrane.

INCUBATION PROCESS

Four conditions are basic to a successful hatch: i) temperature, ii) ventilation, iii) humidity, and iv) position. Using data from extensive tests at the National Agricultural Research Center at Beltsville, MD, poultry scientists have concluded that the optimum incubation temperature is 100°F when the relative humidity is 60 percent, the concentration of oxygen is 21 percent, the carbon dioxide is 0.5 percent, and the air velocity past the eggs is approximately 12 cm (4.75 in) per minute.

TEMPERATURE: The temperature should be as constant and uniform as possible. Instructions provided by the incubator manufacturer should be followed closely. In any case, the temperature at the top of the egg should be 100°F (102°F for still-air incubators.)

HUMIDITY: For a successful hatch, it is necessary to supply moisture to keep the relative humidity about 60 percent during the first 18 days and slightly higher, 70 percent, for the last 3 days. Humidity can be supplied by a pan of water. The water level in the pan must be checked constantly. If humidity needs to be raised, sponges (wicks) may be placed in the pan.

WET-BULB READING IN STILL AIR INCUBATORS

Wet-bulb thermometer readings measure relative humidity in the incubator. The wet-bulb thermometer is encased in a wick-like sock (i.e., hygrometer wick). The wick end is immersed in a reservoir of

TEMPERATURE (°F)	RELATIVE HUMIDITY (%)					
	45	50	55	60	65	70
100	81.3	83.3	85.3	87.3	89.0	90.7
101	82.3	84.2	86.2	88.2	90.0	91.7
102	83.0	85.0	87.0	89.0	91.0	92.7

water. The thermometer cools as water evaporates. The closer the reading between wet and dry thermometers, the higher the humidity. When readings of the two thermometers are equal, the air is saturated.

VENTILATION: Oxygen requirements for gamebird embryos increase rapidly as the embryos develop. To assure adequate oxygen, ventilation with good circulation must be increased as development continues. Temperature and humidity must be adjusted to maintain the correct environment during the increased ventilation.

POSITIONING:: Egg position must be changed at least three to five times daily. An "X" or date marked on one side of the egg and an "O" on the other side will help you keep track when using manual (as opposed to automatic) tray turning.

INCUBATION PERIODS (days)

Canada Goose	35	Peacock	27-28
Ducks:		Pheasant	23-24
Muscovy	33-35	Pigeon	16-18
Other	28	Quail	23-24
Goose	29-31	Swan	42
Guinea	26-28	Turkey	28
Ostrich	42		

HATCHERY SANITATION

The hatchery has long been recognized as a potential source of infection in newly hatched chicks. Causative agents of hatchery-borne diseases are often introduced by contaminated hatching eggs. Hatchery sanitation must include not only the handling of hatching eggs, but the health and management of breeder flocks. Prevention of hatchery-borne disease is the responsibility of all employees — management and workers alike.

Many hatchery problems can be minimized by an effective flow of work in the hatchery. Ventilation, partitioning, building materials, worker traffic, worker clothing, and appropriate worker hygiene all are important. Be alert for common causes of trouble in hatcheries. For instance, shell quality begins to deteriorate during the second year of lay, and penetration by microbes becomes more likely. So aging breeder flocks could be a source of bacterial infections in the hatchery. Aspergillus (fungus) contamination often spreads from the egg and candling room into incubators and ventilation ducts. Staphylococcus and salmonella organisms can be accidentally carried in by plant personnel, farm workers, or visitors.

MANAGEMENT FACTORS

1. Maintain complete health and performance records on each breeder flock.

2. Maintain health records on progeny. Any disease outbreak that implicates the breeder flock or hatchery should be investigated. Records are essential for this purpose.

3. Use young breeding flocks. Shell quality deteriorates in eggs produced by older flocks. Eggs from flocks in their second year of lay should not be used in the hatchery.

4. Practice flock sanitation to assure a supply of clean, safe hatching eggs.

5. Establish a hatchery-wide sanitation program.

   a. Keep all pets and other animals out of hatchery. Control flies and vermin.

   b. Clean, sanitize, and fumigate incubators and hatchers after each set or hatch.

   c. Practice vigilant room sanitation, including periodic inspections and fumigation.

d.   Adopt and enforce a hatchery sanitation inspection program, including monitoring the level of microbial contamination in the air.

e.   Establish and practice in-machine egg-fumigation procedures.

f.   Culture under-grade chicks and pips routinely.

FACILITIES

1.   PLANT LAYOUT — Room and equipment layout should provide a smooth, single-direction flow of eggs from cooler to chick room. Cross-traffic of eggs or employees violates biosecurity.

2.   CONSTRUCTION — The hatchery should have concrete floors, masonry walls, and washable ceilings. Inside walls and partitions should be smooth and solid with tight-fitting doors.

3.   VENTILATION — Egg, setter, hatcher, and chick rooms should have independent ventilation to prevent transport of pathogens to adjacent rooms. Filtered-air-positive-pressure (FAPP) ventilation is desirable for hatcher and chick rooms, where the freshest and safest air is required. Air inlets should be positioned so that expelled air from the building exhausts cannot be reintroduced into the hatchery.

PERSONNEL

1.   Require personnel to be clean and to wear clean, freshly laundered clothing.

2.   Minimize (prohibit, if possible) worker cross-traffic within the hatchery.

3.   Keep unauthorized personnel (visitors, farm help, processing help, business representatives) out of critical areas.

4.   Prohibit food and drink in work areas.

EGGS

1.   Hatch only clean eggs.

2.   If your suppliers cannot provide CLEAN eggs, you will need to wash and sanitize or fumigate eggs in your egg-receiving room.

3.   Hold eggs up to 5 days before placing in the incubator.

HATCHING-EGG SANITATION

The destruction of bacteria on hatching eggs is an important part of hatchery sanitation. Clean eggs should not nor need not be washed. Stained and soiled eggs should be washed and sanitized before being placed into the incubator trays. This can be done manually or with mechanical egg-washing equipment. Water temperature is very important. Always follow manufacturer's instructions on water-temperature settings and washing procedures. Never dip or apply cold water to warm eggs. The wash water temperature (110ºF is the usual recommendation) must be hotter than the egg temperature. The use of commercial egg-washing detergent sanitizer is safe for hatching eggs if used in concentrations recommended.

PRE-INCUBATION FUMIGATION

Routine on-farm fumigation of eggs for hatching will eliminate salmonella infections from poultry flocks. All eggs for hatching should be fumigated. Formaldehyde gas, if used promptly after the eggs are laid, will destroy salmonella organisms on the shell's surface. The procedure requires an inexpensive gas-tight cabinet equipped with fans to circulate the gas during fumigation and to clear the gas afterwards. Eggs for fumigation should be placed on racks so the gas can reach the entire surface. Plastic trays used for washing market eggs are ideal for this purpose.

A high level of formaldehyde gas is obtained by mixing 3 ml of formalin (37% formaldehyde) with 175 mg of potassium permanganate ($KMnO_4$) for each cubic foot of space in the cabinet. An earthenware, galvanized, or glass container holding at least 10 times the volume of the total ingredients should be used for mixing the chemicals. Eggs and fumigant should remain in the cabinet for 20 minutes and the gas then cleared from the cabinet. Humidity for this method of pre-incubation fumigation is not critical, but temperature should be maintained at approximately 70ºF.

Upon placement in the incubator, eggs should be routinely fumigated. Recommendations for loaded-incubator fumigation vary widely with makes and models. Fumigate according to the manufacturer's instructions. Alternate procedures to within-incubator egg fumigation include use of hydrogen peroxide or a germicide called Tek-Trol. Hatchery supply companies can provide information and materials needed.

DRUG USE GUIDE

ACTIVE INGREDIENTS	PRE-SLAUGHTER WITHDRAWAL DAYS	BRAND NAME EXAMPLES
Aklomide	5	Akolomix
Amprolium	0	Amprol
Arsenicals[1]:		
arsanilic acid,	5	Pro-Gen; Roxarsone;
sodium arsanilate		3-Nitroroxarsone
Bacitracin	0	Bacitracin, ZN, MD
Bambermycins	0	Flavomycin, Gainpro
Carbarsone	5	Carb-O-Sep
Ceftiofur sodium (Inject 1D)	21	Naxcel-SP
Chlortetracycline	1	Aureomycin; CTC; Pfichlor
Chlortetracycline	1	Aureomycin soluble powder
Clopidol	0	Coyden-25
Decoquinate	0	Deccox
Erythromycin phosphate	1	Gallimycin 50
Erythromycin(in water)	2	Gallimycin 100
Gentamicin sulfate (inject 1D)	63	Garasol
Halofuginone hydrobromide	7	Stenorol premix
Halofuginone hydrobromide and bambermycins	7	Stenorol + Flavomycin
Halofuginone hydrobromide and virginiamycin	7	Stenorol + Stafac
Hygromycin B	3	Hygromix
Lasalocid sodium	0	Avatec
Lincomycin	0	Lincomix
Manduramicin ammonium	5	Cygro
Monensin[2]	0	Coban 60

[1],[2]See page 28

(CONTINUED)

ACTIVE INGREDIENTS	PRE-SLAUGHTER WITHDRAWAL DAYS	BRAND NAME EXAMPLES
Narasin[3]	0	Monteban
Neomycin	5	Neomycin Sulfate, Neo-terra
Nicarbazin	4	Nicarb
Nitarsone	5	Histostat-50
Nitromide[4]	5	Unistat-3
Novobiocin	4	Albamix
Oxytetracycline	5	Terramycin, OXTC, OTC
Oxytetracycline (injected)	5	Terramycin injectable
Oxytetracycline (in water)	0	Terramycin soluble
Potassium Penicillin G (in water)	1	Potassium Penicillin G USP. grade
Procaine penicillin G and dihydrostreptomycin sulfate (injected)	30	Mycillin-V
Robenidine HCl	5	Robenz
Roxarsone[5]	5	Roxarsone, 3 Nitro
Salinomycin	0	Biocox, Sacox
Sodium Sulfachloropyrazine	4	ESB-3
Spectinomycin HCl Pentahydrate	5	Spectam
Streptomycin sulfate	4	Biotech, Vetstrep
Sulfadimethoxine & ormetoprim	5	Rofenaid
Sulfadimethoxine	5	Albon
Sulfamethazine	10	Sulmet
Sulfanitran & Aklomide	5	Novastat-W
Sulfaquinoxaline	10	Sulfaquinoxaline, SQ
Tetracycline hydrochloride	4	Many brands
Thiabendazole	0	TBZ
Tylosin tartrate (injected)	3	Tylan Injectable
Tylosin tartrate (in water)	1	Tylan Soluble
Tylosin	5	Tylan Premix

[3,4,5]See page 28

(CONTINUED)

ACTIVE INGREDIENTS	PRE-SLAUGHTER WITHDRAWAL DAYS	BRAND NAME EXAMPLES
Virginiamycin	0	Stafac
Zoalene	0	Zoamix

[1]Toxic to waterfowl.
[2]Toxic to equine, adult turkeys, and quail.
[3]Toxic to equine, adult turkeys, and quail.
[4]Toxic to waterfowl
[5]Toxic to waterfowl

Preslaughter withdrawal times listed here for each drug applies to that drug, whether used alone or in combination with other drugs. Combining certain drugs may extend the withdrawal time. Such combinations are listed here. When calculating withdrawal time, each withdrawal day is a full 24 hours, starting with the hour the bird last received the drug.

This listing is neither inclusive or exclusive and in no way constitutes a recommendation, or lack thereof, by the author.

CALCULATING DRUG DOSAGE

Safe and effective administering of drugs and antibiotics requires close and accurate dosages. Drugs and antibiotics can be administered in the feed and water or by parental injection. In gamebirds, most medications are administered in the feed or drinking water. Route of administration may be dependent on the solubility of the drug. Insoluble medications must be administered in the feed. That being the case, be advised that the U.S. Food and Drug Administration (FDA) regulates the approval of drugs that may be legally used with all animals, especially those species grown for food. Drugs administered in the feed must comply with FDA dosage, drug combinations, withdrawal times, and other specific requirements.

Any drug or medicine given in the drinking water must also comply with FDA guidelines as to withdrawal and dose limitations. Putting medicine in the drinking water offers many advantages. Water-administered treatments are easy to start and stop. Sick birds continue to drink even when they are off feed, thus enabling a more rapid response to medication. Most water-dispersible medications are packaged and labeled for water volumes suitable for flocks of commercial-size.

Administration of drinking water medications can be facilitated by "Medicators." Medicators are mechanical devices plumbed into the water line; their function is to meter a measured volume of drug stock (i.e., concentrated) solution into the water lines that supply the water fountains. Most medicators will meter 1/2 to 1 oz stock solution per gallon of drinking water. The concentration of the stock solution must be sufficient to provide the prescribed drug concentration at the final dilution juncture or at the watering fountain. Most gamebird operations are relatively small in relation to commercial poultry flocks, and producers seldom need the drinking water volumes required for commercial production.

For this reason, some calculations are needed to adapt commercially packaged medicinals to small flock or gamebird uses. All drugs should be administered at manufacturer's labeled instructions, based on FDA approved rate. It may be necessary that the user convert US weights and measures to metric weights and measures.

SOLUBLE PREPARATION:

First, check drug label for:

      Required dilution of packet (total gal)

      Packet weight (oz)

      Active drug content (g)

CALCULATION REQUIRED:

Determine water requirement (gal) per oz of drug:

Divide: Total volume (gal) of solution (given on label) by packet
      weight (oz, also from label) = gal/oz of drug.

EXAMPLE:

Packet label calls for 128 gal of water. Packet-weight is 8 oz.

$$128 \text{ gal}/8 \text{ oz} = 16 \text{ gal/oz}$$

LIQUID PREPARATION

Total volume in oz   Total drug in g

EXAMPLE: Dose is 200 mg/gal drinking water

              Drug or ounce = 1 g (1000 mg)/oz

              Divide: mg/oz over dose per gallon = 1000 mg/200 mg
tells you there is 1 oz of liquid drug to 5 gal drinking water (final
dilution 200 mg/gal).

ACCURACY & SAFETY OF ADMINISTERING DRUGS: Mix total contents of
the drug packet into the prescribed volume of water to prepare the
stock (concentrate) solution. Administer daily with liquid measure of
one ounce stock solution per gallon of drinking water. This provides
safety and accuracy of day-to-day medication in the drinking water.

EXAMPLE: One 6-oz packet of medicine to medicate 50 gal of drinking
water.

PREPARE STOCK SOLUTION: Put one 6-oz packet of medicine into
medicator jug. Add 50 oz of water. Dose is 1 oz stock solution per
gallon of drinking water. Mix fresh daily.

DRUGS FOR GAMEBIRDS
SUGGESTED INVENTORY

The wise gamebird grower will habitually be prepared for challenges to the health of the flock. The following listing includes those medications that are most likely to be required in treating health problems.

Those marked with an * are most important. Sufficient dosages for 3 to 5 days' treatment should be retained on hand, or be immediately (i.e., same day) available from your supplier.

As for the other medications listed, they should be accessible within a few days. It may be a good idea to discuss the situation with your supplier, so that there need be no delay in obtaining the medications needed.

Make arrangements for safe storage of your medications, and keep records of their use.

ANTIBIOTICS:

   *Penicillin

   *Gallimycin

   *Tetracyclines (Aureo & Terra)

   *Neomycin

   *Bacitracin

   Tylan

   LS-50

DRUGS:

   *NF180 - NFZ (off the market)

   *Agribon

   Histostat--blackhead prevention

   Other Sulfas -- SQ, Sulmet, etc

COCCIDIOSTATS:

   *Amprol

   *Rofenaid

   Coban [(Monensin, Salinomycin, Lasolocid) Approved for quail but toxic and may cause paralysis. Toxic to Equine.]

COCCIDIOSTATS (CONTINUED):
   Halofuginone (Stenorol)
   Coyden (also antimalarial)

WORMERS (ANTHELMINTICS):

   *Tramisol
   *Safeguard (fenbendazole)/Panacur
   Albendazole (Velbezon)
   Piperazine
   Ivermectin (Cattle)
   TBZ

DRUGS FOR HISTOMONIASIS TREATMENT:

   CAUTION: None of the following are FDA-cleared for Gamebirds. Owner uses at his own risk. Withdraw medication 30
   days before sale or release.

Emtryl — Residual by some producers (Available in Canada)

NF 180/NFZ — Off the market. Helps control the *E. Coli* part of
Blackhead

Flagyl (Metronidazole) — Human drug. Requires prescription.

Histostat (Roxarsone) — Preventive only for feed. Toxic to waterfowl
and dogs.

(New) Albendazole —Velbezon wormer: effective against giardia in
dogs, probably helpful against Histomonas.

(New) Quinocrine (quinine derivative) Anti-malarial. May be toxic
at experimental dog dose [6.6 mg/kg — BID — 5 days]. 100%
effective against Giardia in dogs.

Copper Sulfate — Helpful but not a cure
   In feed 2 #/T/5 days
   In water 1/2000 dilution (1 oz/ 15 gal)

SOURCE —
   Pennsylvania Gamebird Bulletin XXVI: 6. (May/Jun 1994)

GROWER'S REFERENCE

ON

GAMEBIRD HEALTH

II BACTERIAL AND FUNGAL DISEASES — 33

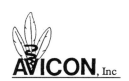

AVICON, Inc

ASPERGILLOSIS

DEFINITION:

Aspergillosis is a fungal disease, usually of the respiratory system, caused by *Aspergillus fumigatus. A. fumigatus* occurs world-wide but was first described in turkeys in 1898. This disease affects gamebirds, wild birds, and domestic poultry. All bird species, mammals, humans, and plants are susceptible. Aspergillosis is characterized by respiratory distress and caseous plaques in lungs and air sacs. Synonyms are brooder pneumonia, mycotic pneumonia, and pneumomycosis. Spores are almost universally present but the disease develops as an on-farm problem and seldom becomes epidemic. Litter materials, especially sawdust and tree bark, are common sources of the fungus. Contaminated ventilation ducts in hatcheries are also Aspergillus-problem areas. Aspergillosis acquired by hatchlings at the hatchery is called brooder pneumonia but when acquired later is called Aspergillosis. Aspergillosis is an environmental disease that does not spread bird-to-bird. When humidity is high, the rate of spread is low. Aspergillosis occurs frequently in captive gamebirds, zoological birds, and domestic poultry. Healthy birds resist infection but can be infected with overwhelming exposure. The incubation period is 4 to 10 days. The course of the acute form of the disease can be as long as 6 weeks, with the chronic form lasting 3 months.

TRANSMISSION AND CLINICAL SIGNS:

Infection usually follows inhalation of large numbers of spores from heavily contaminated feed, litter, or environment. Conjunctival infections may occur from exposure to airborne spores. The disease is not highly contagious. High humidity will reduce the rate of new infections. Acute signs are dyspnea, gasping, sleepiness, loss of appetite, and occasionally paralysis and convulsions. In systemic aspergillosis, the fungus infects the brain and spinal cord. Other signs include tremors, paresis, stunting, anorexia and cyanosis of individual birds. The rate of infection will vary from 2 to 90 percent but is more often in the 5 to 10 percent range. Mortality increases with stress and handling of infected birds. Before death, the birds will gasp, show weakness and incoordination, and die if held upside down. Birds become very uneven in size because of the slow-growth stunting effect on the more severely infected birds. Chronically affected birds exhibit open-mouth breathing because the infection disrupts oxygen-carbon dioxide exchange. Birds have shallow breathing, thus the open mouth.

LESIONS AND DIAGNOSIS:

Hard yellow or gray lesions develop in the respiratory tract especially in the lungs and air sacs. With hatchery-borne aspergillosis (brooder pneumonia) miliary (innumerable) abscesses are in the lungs. Aspergillus lesions of viscera and air sacs are called plaques. Plaques occur at sites where the fungus attaches to the tissue. Exudates and tissue debris form a hard yellow cheesy exudate with a convex/concave (plaque) shape. The fungus is found in the concave surface of the plaque. The signs and gross lesions suggest a diagnosis of aspergillosis. Confirmed diagnosis can be done by microscopic demonstration of the fungus in fresh preparations, laboratory cultures, and histologic tissue sections of the lesions. Laboratory culturing requires 2 to 5 days. Start treatment and control procedures when gross lesions are present.

TREATMENT AND CONTROL:

There is no cure for infected birds; however the flock should be medicated with an antimycotic drug. To control the spread of the disease in the house, increase the humidity, eliminate the source of infection, and medicate the flock with mycostatin. As supplemental treatment, add a fungistat (mold-curb, sodium or calcium propionate or copper sulfate) in the feed or acidified copper in the drinking water for 3 days. Spray the litter lightly with copper sulfate or oil-base germicide to control the dust. In severe outbreaks, litter should be replaced with new bright bark-free shavings or straw. If litter is replaced as a part of the treatment, it should be done before birds are medicated. Copper sulfate is corrosive to metal; therefore, it should be handled in plastic, glass, or ceramic fountains and waterers.

PREVENTION:

Thoroughly clean, disinfect and thermal mist the building between broods. Use only bright clean litter. (Do not use litter materials that have been wet or are moldy.) Do not use shavings that are high in bark content. Spray floors with copper sulfate solution before putting down the new litter. In breeder flocks, collect clean eggs, then sanitize and/or fumigate eggs before setting. Never set eggs that have thin or cracked shells. Follow recommended hatchery C&D program. Clean and sanitize water fountains daily. Use mold inhibitor drugs in the feed. Cull and destroy noticeably infected birds.

AVIAN TUBERCULOSIS

DEFINITION:

Avian tuberculosis (TB) is a chronic, incurable, slow-spreading granulomatous bacterial infection of mature birds characterized by granulomas or tubercles (tumor-like lesions) in the viscera. The birds will
show progressive weight loss, emaciation, and finally death. Synonyms for avian tuberculosis include tuberculosis, TB, and Avian TB.
The causative organism is an acid-fast soil-borne bacterium, *Mycobacterium avium*, that is related to mammalian tuberculosis. The incubation period ranges from months to one or more years.

The bacterium is quite resistant in soil and found in high numbers in
tubercles. Most avian species, including gamebirds, domestic poultry,
songbirds, crows, cranes, parrots, and canaries are susceptible. Avian
TB is highly infectious to swine, occasionally found in bovine but
rarely in humans (the human tuberculosis is caused by *Mycobacterium
tuberculosis*). Avian tuberculosis is reported world-wide but becomes
endemic on premises of small flocks where birds are kept longer than
2 to 3 years. TB is rarely found in commercial poultry flocks.

TRANSMISSION AND CLINICAL SIGNS:

Transmission of the disease is predominately through ingestion of
contaminated feed, water, litter, and soil. Infected birds excrete the
organism in the feces, thus spread within a flock is from bird to environment to bird. Sources of TB dissemination are droppings of wild
birds (pigeon, sparrow, starlings, etc.), contaminated shoes and/or
equipment, and infected feces from swine. Other sources of infection
are from infected dead birds, rodents found in gamebird pens, and
viscera of infected dead pen-mates.

Clinically affected birds are usually older than one year. Disease pro-
gression within the flock is slow, with few noticeably sick birds. Infected birds progressively lose weight, even though they retain their
appetite, and develop diarrhea. TB in the bone produces lameness,
and in late stages, the birds become emaciated and die. Dead birds
show extreme emaciation (consumption).

LESIONS AND DIAGNOSIS:

Internal multiple granulomas or tubercles of varying size and yellowish in color will be found in the liver, spleen, intestines, and/or other
organs. The overall appearance of the bird and the presence of tubercles should alert the pathologist to the probability of TB. Diagnosis is

based on typical flock-farm history, clinical signs, gross lesions of multiple organs and the demonstration of acid-fast bacteria on smears from the tubercles.

When cutting through the tubercles, one will feel a grating effect on the knife. Confirmation of the disease should include identification of the organism from cultures of the tubercles and/or bone marrow. Suspect flocks can be tested by injecting avian tuberculin intradermally on wattle or wing web. Tests are read in 48 hours. Even though the test for avian TB is available, TB testing is seldom done because the procedure is delicate with high risk of bird injury.

TREATMENT AND CONTROL:

Treatment of avian TB is not recommended. Chemotherapy (antibiotics) is ineffective. Control is best managed by depopulating infected and older flocks followed with a thorough C & D of all buildings and indoor pens. Strict sanitization of building and equipment must be carried out before repopulating. Birds should be segregated by age and species; exposure to swine, rabbits, sheep and bovine must be prevented. Rodents (TB carriers) must be eliminated.

PREVENTION:

The key is good sanitation, isolation, and management. Dispose of the infected flock and repopulate with birds from TB-free stock. Initiate proper hygiene and husbandry. Incinerate dead birds. Separate flocks by age and species as well from other animals. Control rodents (infected rodents are often reservoirs of avian TB on poultry and swine farms). Keep breeder birds for no more than two breeding seasons. Gamebirds and poultry older than 2 years are suspect of TB infection. Avian TB in ornamental collections is difficult to eradicate. New additions to collections should be isolated for 2 to 3 months. Avian tuberculosis is prevented with an annual turnover of all gamebirds. This can be achieved by releasing or slaughtering mature birds.

BORDETELLOSIS

DEFINITION:

Bordetellosis is an acute highly contagious upper respiratory disease of young turkeys, quail, and partridge. It is caused by a bacterium and characterized by foamy conjunctivitis, rhinitis, snicking, rales, mucoid nasal exudates, dyspnea, and death. Synonyms include turkey coryza (TC), bordetella rhinotracheitis, and *B. avium*. The cause is *Bordetella avium*, a gram negative nonfermenting motile bacterium. The organism is resistant in the environment, readily cultured from the litter of outbreak flocks, resistant to most antibiotics and drugs, but susceptible to most germicides. Incubation requires 7 to 9 days and the course of the disease is 2 to 6 weeks. Young turkeys and quail, 1 to 6 weeks of age, are the most susceptible. The disease has been reported in most turkey-producing areas of the United States, most European countries, Israel, and South Africa.

A similar disease called Turkey Rhinotracheitis has been reported in England, but unlike Bordetellosis, the disease is caused by a virus. The viral disease has not been reported in gamebirds. A serological survey of wild turkeys in Arkansas showed 95 percent of the birds were positive.

TRANSMISSION AND CLINICAL SIGNS:

Bordetella spreads from building to building or premise to premise by the usual methods that disease spreads. Airborne spread is unlikely. The bacterium is probably carried in on clothing, shoes, and/or equipment.

Once introduced, bordetella spreads bird to bird and bird to environment or environment to bird by feed, water, and/or litter. Drinking water and litter are the most common methods of in-house spread. Older flocks serve as recovered carriers. Contaminated water remaining in the water line will infect replacement flocks. Infection in flocks not yet 10 days of age is indicative of an environmental source of the disease.

Clinical signs are sudden onset, rapid spread, high morbidity and mortality, stunting, and uneven growth. Sick birds are restless, huddle, act chilly, and develop a weak feeble "chirp." The early signs are clear, mucoid nasal discharge, frothy eye exudates, and pasting of eyelids and nostrils. Birds are less active and flip their heads in trying to clear congestion of air passages. As the condition progresses, the head sinuses puff with air as the bird breathes; many birds will develop edema under the jaw. In older birds, tracheal rales continue several weeks after other signs subside and birds remain more susceptible to other infections, especially colibacillosis. Mortality is highest in 10- to 14-day-old birds, but has been recorded as continuing through 5 weeks of age and reaching 15 percent. Recovered flocks remain less thrifty throughout maturity.

LESIONS AND DIAGNOSIS:

Catarrhal rhinitis and hyperemia of the trachea (tracheitis) are the most consistent lesions. Being an upper respiratory disease, the gross and histological lesions are usually limited to the nasal turbinates, sinuses and trachea. Transient eye swelling, edema of throat, mucoid exudates of pharynx, and tracheal collapse (flattened trachea) are observed.

Histological changes vary from shortened cilia, patchy to complete deciliation, and loss of tracheal mucosa. Exudates consisting of sloughed cells, mucus, and pus cells (heterophils) are present. The immune competency is compromised so birds are more susceptible to other infections. The diagnosis relies heavily on history, clinical signs, lesions, and isolation of the organism, *Bordetella avium*. Cultures should be taken from the nose, sinuses, palatine cleft, and trachea. Serological tests are useful for monitoring recovered and/or other flocks on the premises. Antibiotic sensitivity tests should be requested on isolates from each case. *B. avium* should be suspected in any respiratory disease of gamebirds.

TREATMENT AND CONTROL:

Bordetella is resistant to most medications. Even so, the flock should be medicated according to antibiotic-sensitivity results. In warm seasons, move the flock outdoors or increase ventilation. Also administer supplemental therapy of fortified feeds and vitamins with electrolytes in the drinking water. Wash and sanitize waterers daily. Use iodine water sanitizer [12 to 25 ppm] in the drinking water after medications are discontinued. Fogging the room with tetracycline is reported to reduce clinical signs, but has little benefit in the long term. Vaccines are commercially available and are recommended as part of the treatment and control program.

PREVENTION:

Eradication is the best prevention. Initiate good husbandry and biosecurity. Bordetella eradication requires depopulating, cleaning, disinfecting, and heat fogging of the building, flushing water lines with strong chlorine solution [2 oz/gal], cleaning and sanitizing feed line and bin. Rest the building at least 30 days before repopulating. Eradication may have to be scheduled after the last hatch for the season. Screen out free-flying birds, control traffic patterns for bird care, and use separate caretaker per building, flock, or age group. Vaccines should not be used in an eradication program. When vaccines are used for one or more seasons, the total eradication procedure should follow the last vaccinated flock.

BOTULISM

DEFINITION:

Botulism is an acute intoxication due to ingestion of toxins produced by a bacterium. The disease is characterized by weakness, prostration, flaccid paralyzed neck, and death. Synonyms are limberneck, bulbar paralysis, western duck disease, and alkali disease. The cause is a neurotoxin produced by *Clostridium botulinum*, a spore-forming gram positive anaerobic bacterium. Botulism's incubation requires only a few hours and the course of the disease 4 to 24 hours. Several types of toxins are produced, but types **A**, **C**, and **E** affect birds. The toxin is extremely potent. The minimum lethal dose is 0.00012 mg/kg body weight subcutaneously. The toxin is relatively heat-stable. Botulism in gamebirds usually results from pen mates feeding on decaying carcasses and/or maggots from those carcasses. The bacterium lives in the soil and prefers an alkaline environment characteristic of shallow-flood areas in alkaline soils. All bird species of all ages are susceptible. Type **C** toxin is found world-wide; types **A** and **C** are associated with poultry outbreaks and type **E** is associated with botulism deaths in migratory waterfowl of Canada, western USA, and the Great Lakes area. Type **C** toxin would be the most likely group associated with botulism in upland gamebirds.

TRANSMISSION AND CLINICAL SIGNS:

Botulism is contracted primarily by eating food or decaying matter containing the pre-formed toxin. Decomposing bird carcasses on poultry ranges, wet litter or other organic matter, and maggots from decaying material may contain the toxin. There is no spread bird to bird. There is a possibility of toxin forming in the digestive tracts of birds on high protein diets. In waterfowl, the disease is found in shallow lakes and marshes laden with decaying vegetation, dead fish, and dead invertebrates.

Clinical signs include paralysis within a short time following ingestion. Legs and wings become paralyzed, then the neck becomes limp. Neck feathers may become loose as feather follicles are affected. In lesser doses, signs may be more gradual with drowsiness, weakness, progressive paralysis of legs, wings, and neck. Paralyzed birds may close eyes and seem to be in a coma as the nictitating membrane (third eyelid) becomes paralyzed.

LESIONS AND DIAGNOSIS:

There are no visible or gross lesions. Live birds exhibit paralysis of wings, legs, and neck. Necropsy findings include loose neck feathers, decayed material and/or maggots in crop, proventriculus, and gizzard; and mucus accumulation in the mouth (bird is unable to swallow). When death is prolonged, such birds may exhibit mild enteritis. Botulism must be differentiated from other causes of paralysis such as mycotoxicosis and encephalitic diseases. Diagnosis takes into account the case history, clinical signs, and lesions. Paralysis of the nictitating membrane is diagnostic. Diagnostic procedures include injection of serum from affected birds into mice. High serum toxin levels will kill mice in two to twelve hours. Administer botulism antitoxin to paralytic birds and, if effective, birds will recover in 12 to 24 hours. To further confirm botulism, feed the contents from crop, stomach and gizzard to susceptible birds or laboratory mice and observe for paralysis.

FINAL CONFIRMATION TEST: CHALLENGE - Inject 0.5 ml serum from paralyzed bird abdominally into each of two mice. CONTROL - mix 1.2 ml of suspect serum with 0.3 ml botulism antitoxin. Let set 30 minutes then inject 0.75 ml into each of two additional mice. Death in the Challenge and no death in Control mice constitute a positive test.

TREATMENT AND CONTROL:

Remove spoiled or decaying feed as well as collect and dispose of dead birds to limit the outbreak. Flush flock with Epsom salts [1 lb/2000 birds] in drinking water or wet mash. It has been reported that potassium permanganate [1:3000] in drinking water is helpful. Remove affected birds from flock to a sick pen and treat them with intramuscular or subcutaneous injections of botulism antitoxin. The dose for ducks, turkeys and pheasants is 2 to 4 cc per bird; repeat if needed 12 hours later. Wild ducks can be inoculated in the abdominal cavity. A polyvalent antiserum (Types A and C) is preferred but type C is usually given. Birds having ingested sublethal doses of the toxin usually recover from the flock treatment with access to fresh feed and water. Segregating affected birds from the pen stops the risk of cannibalism by pen mates.

PREVENTION:

Avoid botulism by preventing the access of gamebirds to the source of toxin — promptly removing dead birds, decayed organic material, moldy feed, etc. Incinerate or bury dead birds promptly. DO NOT FEED

SPOILED CANNED VEGETABLES TO BIRDS OR OTHER ANIMALS. Control flies. Fly maggots on botulism carcasses carry high doses of toxin. Add mold inhibitor to feed and replace suspect feed. For wild birds, keep waterfowl away from affected wet areas by draining. Notify Fish and Wildlife Officials when wild birds are involved. Treat the soil where dead birds are found with soil acidifier — e.g., aluminum sulfate, sodium bisulfite, or similar product used for acid-loving landscape plants.

CAMPYLOBACTERIOSIS

DEFINITION:

A contagious bacterial infection found primarily in gamebirds, chickens, turkeys, mammals, and humans. Clinical infection in chickens is characterized by drop in production, and increase in morbidity and mortality. The causal agent, a common intestinal bacterium, is *Campylobacter fetus* subspecies *jejuni*. This agent was formerly named Vibrio and can be cultured on laboratory media or in chicken embryos. However, the bacterium is gram negative, motile, and microaerophilic, and rather resistant to most environmental factors and to many disinfectants. The common names for the disease are vibrionic hepatitis and Campylobacter hepatitis. The incubation period requires 5 to 15 days, and the course of the disease is 3 weeks to termination of the flock.

Of the gamebird species, the wild turkey is the most susceptible to the disease but Campylobacteriosis should always be considered in any gamebird species when hepatitis is the predominant lesion. The disease has been reported in North America and Europe.

> SPECIAL NOTE: Campylobacteriosis has been associated with serious enteric infections in humans. Poultry products have been implicated as a possible source for this type of food poisoning.

TRANSMISSION AND CLINICAL SIGNS:

Campylobacter fetus jejuni is eliminated in feces and spreads to other birds through contaminated feed and water. Infected birds shed the organism for weeks or months. Transmission through the egg is suspected, but has not been proven. Stress factors are thought to precipitate repeat outbreaks of Campylobacter in recovered carrier birds.

Infection in chickens is usually subclinical and confined to the intestine; thus the onset of outbreaks is usually slow and insidious. Morbidity is low at any given time. The numbers of cull birds progressively increase. Infected birds are pale, anemic, thin, unthrifty, and some have jaundice, diarrhea, and dirty dry scaly combs, Acute mortality is low but cumulative mortality is high. Breeder hens lay fewer eggs, strongly impacting total flock performance for the season.

LESIONS AND DIAGNOSIS:

Chronically ill birds are thin, pale, and unthrifty. The most dramatic lesions may involve only the liver. The bone marrow may be pale and watery. Older birds exhibit hemorrhage and necrotic changes in the liver lesions that vary from gross swelling to large necrotic areas. The spleen and kidneys are commonly affected. Young birds frequently will have catarrhal enteritis. Other lesions include ascites, hydropericardium, and cardiomyopathy or myocardial flabbiness. The diagnosis is strongly based on history, typical gross and histological lesions and isolation of the causative bacterium. Intestinal distention accompanies the enteric or diarrheic form.

The Campylobacter organism can be isolated on blood agar media or by yolk-sac inoculation of 5- to 8-day-old chicken embryos. When the embryo dies, the bacteria can be demonstrated in stained yolk smears or subcultures on blood agar media. The bile is a reservoir for this agent; therefore cultures should be made from the bile. Tissues for culturing include liver, bile, spleen, kidney, ascitical fluids, heart, intestine, and cloacal contents. Keep culture samples moist.

TREATMENT AND CONTROL:

Treatment is not very satisfactory. Drugs used for treatment may also be used in prevention programs. Dihydrostreptomycin, which is essentially removed from the market, is usually effective. Furazolidone, if available, is beneficial but must be administered in the feed. Most strains of Campylobacter confer little or no immunity. There is no effective vaccine. Either penicillin or gallimycin (erythromycin) will reduce the mortality. Therapy with tetracycline, lincomycin, and spectinomycin offers some benefit but is not a cure. Flock mortality tends to be higher than normal for the duration of the flock. DO NOT SAVE BIRDS FROM INFECTED FLOCKS FOR FUTURE BREEDING BIRDS!

PREVENTION:

Eradication, probably the best and only reliable form of prevention, requires flock depopulation followed by thorough cleaning and disinfecting of facilities and equipment. DO NOT CARRY OVER BIRDS FROM INFECTED FLOCKS. Select a different breed or strain of replacement birds, seeking birds of breeds that show some resistance to this disease. Upgrade the general flock hygiene, biosecurity, and other husbandry practices to control other diseases and parasites. Never add birds to a started flock.

Broad-spectrum antibiotics are beneficial in the health and well being of the birds as they help control of other infections. The bottom line is good biosecurity, known good management, and good husbandry.

CANDIDIASIS

DEFINITION:

Candidiasis is a disease affecting gamebirds and domestic poultry. The disease is caused by a yeast-like fungus, characterized by whitish raised areas in the crop, proventriculus, erosions in the gizzard and inflammation of the vent area. The common names are thrush (crop) and vent gleet (inflammation), and a former name was Moniliasis. The causative agent is *Candida albicans*. Incubation period is 7 to 21 days and the course of the disease is long and chronic. The preferred culture media is Sabouraud dextrose agar with chloramphenicol and cycloheximide. The colonies grow to 1/4 inch in diameter and smell like baker's yeast.

Poor sanitation and overuse of antibiotics contribute to the problem. Birds of all ages are susceptible. Candidiasis has been reported in all the common pen-raised gamebird species. Humans and domestic animals are also susceptible. This disease occurs worldwide in poultry-producing areas, especially in caged- and confinement-rearing systems.

TRANSMISSION AND CLINICAL SIGNS:

Infection results from ingestion of the Candida organism in contaminated feed and water. The disease does not spread directly from bird to bird, but rather from bird to feed and/or water trough to bird. *C. albicans* grows readily in unsanitary water troughs, hence the source of spread. This fungus also grows on feed grains, thus moldy lumpy feed is often the introductory source into a gamebird flock.

The disease is primarily of the digestive tract of birds. The organism is often present in the normal digestive tract of the healthy bird; if some other debilitating condition develops, pathological Candidiasis lesions may appear. There are no specific clinical signs, but infected birds become pale or anemic, are listless, unthrifty, retarded in growth, and show dry ruffled feathers. Birds with vent gleet will have diarrhea and soiled vent feathers and whitish encrustation on posterior extremities. The young are more seriously affected than mature birds.

LESIONS AND DIAGNOSIS:

Gross lesions are confined mostly to the crop, stomach, and gizzard. In severe cases lesions also develop in the mouth and esophagus. Intestinal infection accompanies these conditions, but without the presence of descriptive lesions. The crop lesions are focal thickenings, i.e., circular, whitish, and raised areas. The term of "terry-cloth effect" is used to describe crop lesions.

Proventriculus and gizzard lesions are "erosions" of the mucosa and the lining. The intestinal form is commonly a mucocatarrhal enteritis. Vent gleet tends to accompany the enteritis form of the infection. A presumptive diagnosis can be rendered on the basis of gross lesions. A wet-mount crop smear that demonstrates "yeast-like" organisms further supports the diagnosis.

Confirmatory diagnosis is based on the isolation and identification of the organism. The preferred laboratory media is Sabouraud dextrose agar. The yeast cells develop glossy white colonies that emit the odor of baker's yeast.

TREATMENT AND CONTROL:

Flock medication with antimycotic drugs will usually control the infection. Effective medicinals include nystatin (an antibiotic), products with copper-copper sulfate, and acidified copper. Commercially prepared products should be used according to label instructions. Copper sulfate can be used in the drinking water at 1:2000 dilution [1 oz/16 gal of water] or in the feed [1 to 2 lb/ ton]. Products with copper should be used for only 3 days, as prolonged use of copper leads to copper toxicity in poultry and ruminant animals. For this reason, litter and manure cannot be disposed of on lands where ruminants graze. Dispose of these materials on cultivated land. Since copper sulfate is corrosive to galvanized metals, copper compounds can be safely administered only in nonmetalic containers. Nystatin, an antifungal antibiotic, must be used in the feed for 7 to 14 days.

Other control measures focus on daily cleaning and sanitization of watering troughs and fountains and reduced use of antibiotics.

PREVENTION:

Lax management practices contribute to candidiasis. Prevention requires correction, namely daily cleaning and sanitization of watering troughs and fountains and addition of sanitizers to the drinking water; prompt removal of wet litter; addition (during manufacture) of mold-inhibiting drugs to feed; regular clean-outs of the feed bins (to remove lumpy feed). Mold-inhibiting drugs include propionic acid, and sodium or calcium propionate and are added to the feed when manufactured. Water sanitizers include chlorine coninuously and iodine solutions 3 to 4 days per week. Continuous chlorine [3 to 5 ppm] can be added to the drinking water.

NOTE: Prepare a **stock solution** by mixing water and Clorox [1 1/2 oz Chlorox/1 gal of water]. Add 1 oz of this **stock solution** to each gal of the flock's drinking water to achieve the desired level of 3 to 5 ppm continuous medication.

Administer the iodine [12 to 25 ppm] for 3 to 4 days per week. Iodine tends to foam thus hampering normal function of medicator machine. The use of these guidelines will minimize the incidence of Candidiasis.

CHLAMYDIOSIS

DEFINITION:

Chlamydiosis, an acute to chronic contagious disease of wild and domestic birds, is characterized by intestinal, respiratory, or systemic infections. The disease is transmissible to other animals and humans and in most states is classified as a "reportable disease." Synonyms include ornithosis, psittacosis, and parrot fever. Initially it was named for the source, psittacosis from psittacine (curved beaked) or ornithosis from ornithine (straight-beaked) birds.

Today, veterinarians refer to the disease as Chlamydiosis. The causative organism is *Chlamydia psittaci*, a virus-like organism. *C. psittaci* is an obligate intracellular bacterium. All strains contain an identical genus-specific antigen. Infected tissue cells contain red staining bodies (Chlamydia organisms). Incubation requires 5 to 7 days, and the course of the disease is acute to chronic over a long time. Virulence varies with strain.

The organism multiplies in the respiratory epithelium. *Chlamydia psittaci* can be grown in chicken embryo and in cell cultures from chicken, mouse, and guinea pig. Turkeys, psittacine birds, pigeons, ducks, many other bird species, humans, and certain animal species are susceptible. Younger birds are most susceptible. The disease occurs world-wide and is prevalent in wild colony-nesting species.

TRANSMISSION AND CLINICAL SIGNS:

Transmission is primarily by inhalation of fecal dust. Can be bird to bird, feces to bird, and bird to man via contaminated clothing and equipment. CHLAMYDIA IS NOT EGG PASSED. Recovered birds remain carriers and shedders for 42 days or longer. Environmental stress may provoke a reoccurrence of frank disease in carrier birds. The more-virulent strains affect gulls, egrets, turkeys, and some psittacines; the less-virulent strains are found in pigeons, ducks, and psittacines.

Early clinical signs include depression, loss of appetite, respiratory distress, and loose yellow to yellow-green droppings. Signs in infected turkeys include nasal-ocular discharge, conjunctivitis, weakness, inappetence, weight loss, diarrhea, and death. Infected turkeys may also rest with point of sternum (keel) on the ground, reducing pressure on the painful abdomen. Ornithine birds develop diarrhea followed by death; psittacine birds the same but psittacines may also have brain hemorrhage; humans develop headaches, fever to 104°F, and pneumonia-like symptoms.

When Chlamydiosis is diagnosed in the flock and human illness follows, a physician should be notified. The illness might be psittacosis, i.e., the human form of this disease.

LESIONS AND DIAGNOSIS:

Airsacculitis, pericarditis, perihepatitis, and peritonitis with serofibrinous exudate, focal necrosis of liver and spleen, liver and spleen enlargement, and fibrinous pneumonia are gross lesions found in the acute stage of the disease. Lesions found in chronic form include swollen liver and spleen as well as discoloration of the liver. Lesions may be absent in the infected, but inapparent, carrier or shedder bird.

A tentative diagnosis and treatment can be based on the described gross lesions. Absolute confirmation requires isolation and identification of the organism, a laboratory procedure that takes up to 14 days in chicken embryos or mice. The presence of cytoplasmic inclusions in tissue smears and histological tissue sections is confirmatory. Serological and other cultural procedures are needed to differentiate the infection from other known systemic and respiratory diseases, such as mycoplasma, fowl cholera, and colibacillosis.

TREATMENT AND CONTROL:

Chlamydiosis occurs sporadically in poultry. An effective vaccine is not available. The disease responds well to chlortetracycline (CTC/aureomycin) therapy at the rate of 200 to 400 g/ton of feed for 3 weeks. Initial medication [400 mg/gal] can be given in the drinking water until the flock is receiving the medicated feed. Other antibiotics are less effective, and therefore not recommended. Seed-eating aviary birds should be treated with CTC-impregnated seed [0.5 mg/g]. Treat fruit- and nectar-eating birds by adding CTC [0.5 mg/ml] to nectar for 30 to 45 days. Do not release and market gamebirds until full treatment period has been completed. Recovered birds are safe for processing. Federal Drug Administration (FDA) withdrawal period for the respective medication is 2 days. Outbreaks should be reported to regulatory and Public Health Officials.

PREVENTION:

Good management by isolation, proper hygiene, and strict biosecurity are the best methods of prevention. Restrict visitors' access to pens, prevent exposure to other animals, do not mix birds of different species and ages. Screen wild birds from brooding-rearing facilities.

COLIBACILLOSIS

DEFINITION:

Colibacillosis is a noncontagious infectious disease of primarily immature gamebirds and poultry caused by pathogenic *Escherichia coli*, a coliform bacterium. This disease is characterized by septicemia, fibrinous exudates and/or granulomas, tumor-like nodules. Synonyms include *E. coli*, EC, Hjarres' disease, and coli septicemia. The causative agent is usually *E. coli* but can include other intestinal or coliform bacteria. Birds of all ages, especially the very young and immune-suppressed, are susceptible to the infection. Disease resistance is impaired in birds exposed to immune-debilitating infections, stress from handling, and acute respiratory infections. The incubation period is 2 to 3 days and the course of the disease is 2 to 6 weeks. Coliform bacteria are found worldwide; the disease will occur anywhere and anytime that bird pens become filthy and overall sanitation becomes substandard. This is a disease of birds living in excrement and filth.

TRANSMISSION AND CLINICAL SIGNS:

Colibacillosis is an environmentally borne disease. Birds become infected by contact with damp, dirty litter and filthy pen conditions. It does not spread bird-to-bird. The signs of illness include unthriftiness, dry dirty ruffled feathers, decreased appetite, depression, diarrhea, and death. Birds become pale and anemic, followed by dirty feathers and pasting around the vent.

LESIONS AND DIAGNOSIS:

Enteritis, diarrhea, and generalized septicemia are the prevalent lesions. Certain birds will exhibit pericarditis and airsacculitis especially following immune-suppressing (usually viral) infections. In the chronic phase of the disease, peritonitis is common. Adult female birds will exhibit salpingitis and uterine infections. The coligranulomas (Hjarres') are tumor-like granulomatous lesions that develop on liver, intestines, or lungs in birds following outbreaks of Histomoniasis (Blackhead). Granulomas can occur in or on any organ and may be confused for avian tuberculosis. Flock history, symptoms, and lesions provide a tentative diagnosis but confirmation requires isolating and identifying the coliform bacteria. Certain serotypes of *E. coli* are consistently pathogenic. The pathogenic isolate usually contains cell-wall structures called "pili." Serotyping procedures require extra laboratory tests, usually for an additional fee. In serious endemic outbreaks, the gamebird grower is advised to request serotyping of the isolate as the isolate would be available to produce an autogenous bacterin if needed.

TREATMENT AND CONTROL:

Treatment must start with improving sanitation of environment, including feeders and waterers. Then administer medication known to be effective against the isolate. Drugs normally helpful include the tetracyclines (aureomycin and terramycin), neomycin, streptomycin, novobiocin, sulfas, and gentamycin. Follow manufacturer's dosage instruction. Medications should be administered for 3 to 5 days. Medication in the drinking water is often the route of choice because of ease of starting and ceasing drug administration. In recurrent endemic farm problems the use of the autogenous bacterin is recommended. Control of Colibacillosis lies in good management and biosecurity.

PREVENTION:

Cleanliness is said to be next to godliness; therefore, strict attention must be directed toward cleanliness and sanitation. This attention must include hatching, egg-gathering, egg-cleaning and storing; the incubator and hatchers, and finally the brooding-rearing facilities. Occasionally, Colibacillosis is traced to free-flying birds that roost over or in gamebird pens. In this case, bird-proof the indoor pens.

ERYSIPELAS

DEFINITION:

Erysipelas is an acute septicemic disease of most species of birds. Characteristics of the disease are cyanosis, purplish areas on the skin, swollen snood (in turkeys), and hemorrhage on muscle and viscera. The causative agent is *Erysipelothrix insidiosa (rhusiopathiae)*. Erysipelas means "red skin" and in humans is called "erysipeloid." The organism is a gram positive, slender, slightly bent pleomorphic nonspore-forming rod, resistant in the environment (especially in alkaline soils) and to many germicides.

The organism grows on laboratory media and in the yolk sac of chicken embryos. The incubation period is 2 to 3 days and the course of the disease is 2 to 4 weeks. Gamebirds, domestic poultry, migratory wildbirds, rodents, large animals (especially swine), and humans are susceptible to erysipelas. The disease is found in semimature to mature birds on dirt-floor buildings or outdoor pens. This disease is common worldwide. In the USA, the disease becomes a problem mostly in the cool months of fall, winter, and spring.

TRANSMISSION AND CLINICAL SIGNS:

Erysipelas is a soil-borne disease in which infected premises are considered the primary source of infection. The infection can readily be introduced on to a premise on shoes, clothing, or equipment contaminated while visiting infected flocks or swine.

Actual infection comes from ingestion of the organism or its entry through mucus membranes or breaks in the skin. The beak and toe nails become contaminated from the soil. It is thought that birds become infected through cannibalism, fighting, foot pad punctures, and mating injuries that would inoculate the organism into the skin of other birds. Experimentally, the disease was spread from sick mice to pigeon by biting insects. Other reports list fish meal as a probable source for poultry. Erysipelas does not spread bird to bird with casual contact. Birds in pens adjacent to sick pens do not become infected.

The organism has been isolated from the semen of male turkeys, therefore, mating and/or insemination is a probable transmission route. At the onset of the disease a few dead birds will be found. Sick birds have swollen joints, are listless and unsteady, and have yellow-green diarrhea. Other signs are birds with skin lesions, loss of appetite and painful movement (arthritic form). Birds will have facial swelling and labored breathing from exudates in air passages. The disease progresses from the acute to the chronic form. Mortality ranges from 2 to 25 percent depending on when medication is initiated. In flocks that are in production, production drops to a level that correlates with the rate of very sick hens or hens that die. Crippled birds with swollen joints are judged to have a chronic infection.

LESIONS AND DIAGNOSIS:

The primary gross lesions are purple-colored skin splotches (cyanosis), catarrhal enteritis, swollen joints, swollen snood (turkey), and dark swollen and congested liver. Other lesions may include enlarged spleen; hydropericardium with endocarditis (inflammation of the heart lining); diffuse hemorrhages in muscles, organs, and tissues; thickened proventriculus; yellow nodules in ceca; and generalized vascular engorgement. Asymptomatic carriers are usually free of gross lesions.

A presumptive diagnosis can be based on the lesions described. However Erysipelas must be differentiated from fowl cholera, staphlylococcosis, streptococcosis, and other acute septicemic diseases. Confirmation requires isolating and identifying the organism in cultures of affected organs or bone marrow. Typical colonies will grow on blood agar in 24 to 48 hours. If erysipelas is endemic on the premises, flock medication should be initiated on the basis of on the presumptive diagnosis. The disease responds dramatically to erysipelas-sensitive antibiotics and the mortalities will subside within 24 to 36 hours. Flock improvement upon medication is evidence supportive of the diagnosis.

TREATMENT AND CONTROL:

Penicillin is the antibiotic of choice since all Erysipelas isolates tend to be sensitive to this antibiotic. Medication can be administered in the feed, water, or both. If medication by feed is immediately available, mix penicillin [100 g/ton] in the feed for 5 to 7 days. If feed medication is not immediately available, mix soluble penicillin in the drinking water [100 mg (1 to 1.5 million units)/gal] for 3 to 5 days or until medicated feed is available. Water and feed medication should overlap no more than 24 to 36 hours. Total medication time should be 5 to 7 days.

Valuable individual birds can be treated with penicillin by injection. Daily or every-other-day injections for at least three injections is recommended. Dosage should be according to instructions on the label.

Medicated birds should not be released for hunting or for slaughter or for human consumption until 7 days following completion of treatment. The use of the bacterin will immunize birds for carry-over for spring or breeder replacements, but a bacterin should be for short-time use or as an interim procedure.

Penicillin therapy is for emergency use so the antibiotic should be on inventory, but management is the only solution for long-term control. Do not mix birds of different ages or species. Keep birds away from mammals. Upgrading basic sanitation and overall flock hygiene and biosecurity will minimize risk of relapse or future outbreaks. Producer awareness and sound management decisions are the best control.

PREVENTION:

Preventive measures are the instructions outlined above in CONTROL. Control is implemented as follow-up to an outbreak, and prevention is the follow-up to control. If gamebirds are maintained on swine premises, one must be prepared for periodic outbreaks. Good management and prudent biosecurity prevent outbreaks. In management, segregate gamebirds by species and age. Keep the flock away from animals.

Biosecurity measures include sanitized boots, clothing, and head gear. Control personnel traffic. The importance of careful C&D (cleaning and disinfecting) of pens cannot be over-emphasized. Preferred disinfectants are compounds containing one or a combination of phenol, creosol, iodine, formaldehyde, and lye. Lye is considered most effective but requires extreme caution for safe use. The applicator must wear protective clothing and indoor facilities must be well-rinsed before birds can safely be placed in the pens.

FOWL CHOLERA

DEFINITION:

Fowl Cholera, one of the oldest known diseases of poultry, was first studied in 1736. Fowl Cholera (FC) is a widely distributed contagious septicemic bacterial disease of most avian species characterized by high morbidity and mortality with extensive hemorrhage and septicemic (blood poison) changes. Acute form is followed by a localized chronic form. Common names are avian pasteurellosis, FC, cholera, and avian hemorrhagic septicemia. The infectious agent is a bacterium, *Pasteurella multocida*, a small gram negative, nonmotile nonspore forming, bipolar rod occurring singly, in pairs, and occasionally in chains. Incubation period is 3 to 9 days. The course of the disease is 2 weeks or until flock is depopulated. There are three or more strains, varying in pathogenicity. The encapsulated strains are highly virulent. The organism will survive several months in soil, litter, or decaying organic matter but is easily killed by disinfectants, drying, and direct sunlight. Epidemic outbreaks have been reported in gamebirds, wild water fowl, domestic poultry, coturnix quail, zoological collections, and aviaries. FC usually strikes birds older than 6 weeks. Recovered birds remain carriers and harbor the organism in their nasal clefts and air passages. In most of the world, FC is commonly reported as sporadic outbreaks, primarily in warm and temperate climates but it does prevail in fall and winter.

TRANSMISSION AND CLINICAL SIGNS:

FC introduction occurs from a variety of sources such as flock additions, free-flying birds, raccoons, rodents, and cats or other animals. Within the pen the organism is spread from birds dead from the disease and cannibalism of sick and dying birds. Scavenging of dead birds by other animals will disseminate the disease to other pens, farms, etc. Contaminated crates, feed bags, shoes and clothing are common sources of spread by caretakers. The infection usually enters the tissues through the mucus membranes of the larynx or upper respiratory tract but the eye and superficial wounds (animal bites) are probable routes of infections of the individual bird. Contamination of feed and water with infected feces and exudates increases disease spread within the pen. The first sign of trouble may be sudden bird deaths and high increase in daily mortality. Outward signs of sick birds are fever, depression, anorexia, mucoid exudates of mouth and nose, yellow-green diarrhea, and increased water consumption. Later, birds lose weight, become lame, and develop rales (rattling in respiratory tract). Dead and dying birds are very cyanotic. Mortality increases logarithmically. Several birds might develop neurological signs and some species develop sinusitis.

LESIONS AND DIAGNOSIS:

Internal lesions vary considerably but typical septicemic changes are present. These include hemorrhage, congestion, and reddening of the tissues, especially the heart, body fats, peritoneum, and mucous membranes. Liver, spleen, and kidneys are swollen, congested, and dark, often with petechial hemorrhages and focal (pin-point) necrosis. In turkeys and related species, pneumonia with lung "consolidations" is common. Consolidated lungs will not float, which is an accurate diagnostic feature. No other pneumonia of birds causes lung consolidation. Meningitis and encephalitis with torticollis (head over back) develop in a few of the infected birds. Dehydration and cyanosis of head and unfeathered parts and dark swollen congested hemorrhagic liver (corn-meal liver) are other diagnostic lesions of the disease. A presumptive diagnosis considers a history of unexplained sudden deaths of adult birds especially with a record of fowl cholera on the premises. Typical or diagnostic lesions are helpful but confirmation requires isolation and identification of the organism from various tissues and/or blood. Impression smears of liver, heart or blood of septicemic cases often reveal bipolar, gram negative bacteria (rods). Laboratory confirmation requires 3 to 5 days. Lung consolidation, along with other lesions of acute septicemia with hemorrhages throughout the carcass, is the reason for calling the condition "hemorrhagic septicemia." Cholera must be differentiated from other acute septicemic diseases. Flock medication should be started on basis of presumptive diagnosis.

TREATMENT AND CONTROL:

Early flock medication is essential to minimize mortality. Sulfonamides, especially sulfadimethoxine (SDM), sulfaquinoxaline (SQ), and sulfamethazine (sulmet) are very effective in stopping and controlling mortality. SDM is the drug of choice because of its lower toxicity to birds. SDM can be administered in the feed or drinking water. Water treatment is preferred for treating acute outbreaks, to be followed by medication in the feed. SDM by way of water is 1/2 oz/gal for 2 to 3 days, then reduced to 0.5 oz/2 gal for 3 more days. The other sulfas would be the same dosage but treatments must be interrupted to accomodate a schedule of 3 days on, 2 days off, 2 days on, 2 off, 2 on, then off. Feed levels would be for the use of "coccidiostat prevention" and can be continued indefinitely. The sulfonamides will lower egg fertility; therefore, medication for birds in production will need to be altered. Also there is a 10-day withdrawal required for birds for release or slaughter. Tetracycline antibiotics have efficacy against Pasteurella, the cholera agent. So this offers a safe alternative for follow-up or supplemental treatment to sulfonamides. Control is best accomplished by prevention with emphasis on eradication as early as feasible, possibly at the end of the season or before the start of a new season. Eradication will require the depopulation of buildings and pens, thorough C & D, pens empty for 2 to 3 months, effective rodent-predator control, and improved biosecurity.

PREVENTION:

Pasteurella multocida is not transmitted through the egg. Prevention requires long-term planning with a program designed around eradication of the disease as well as to avoid its reintroduction. Inactivated vaccines can be used to immunize replacements or carry-over birds. Two inoculations of the vaccine, at 2- to 4-week intervals, are needed for adequate protection. A third inoculation is recommended for breeder birds before the onset of the next production year. Do not use the live-cholera vaccines.

As emphasized above, rodent control is essential to prevent cholera in birds in outdoor pens. Raccoon, skunk, opossum, etc. are common carriers and sources of fowl cholera in birds on range. Isolation and segregation of infected birds or carrier animals are logical preventive procedures. Purchase replacement birds from a FC-clean source. Never add carrier birds to a clean flock. Keep dead birds removed and properly disposed of by burning or burying and away from scavengers, including dogs and cats.

FOWL TYPHOID

DEFINITION:

Fowl typhoid is a contagious egg-transmitted infectious bacterial disease of gamebirds and poultry, characterized by acute and chronic phases, with most of the epidemiological features of Pullorum disease. The disease must be reported to regulatory agencies. The causal agent is *Salmonella gallinarum*, closely related to *S. pullorum*, the non-motile bacterium first reported in England in 1889. Its incubation period is 4 to 5 days; its acute phase lasts 5 to 6 days, and its chronic phase continues for several weeks. The cell-wall antigen is identical to that of *S. pullorum*, thus the pullorum test used for replacement breeder birds will also detect fowl typhoid. Gamebirds, poultry, waterfowl, and wild birds of all ages are susceptible. For this reason, all captive birds on the premises should be tested for pullorum-typhoid. Losses of 40 to 50 percent have been reported.

S. gallinarum is present worldwide, wherever gamebirds and poultry are grown. The disease has been nearly eradicated in the United States, but is still present and difficult to control in Latin American and other developing countries. Sporadic outbreaks can occur in spring and summer. Recent outbreaks have been in the fancier or exotic fowl.

TRANSMISSION AND CLINICAL SIGNS:

Transmission is the same as with pullorum, including passage from infected breeder hen (the carrier) to the chick in the egg.

The disease also spreads among penmates (i.e., bird to bird). The organism is shed in the feces, thus spread through contaminated feed, water, and litter is common. Infected birds are unthrifty, droopy and listless; show ruffled feathers, pale combs and/or facial tissues; and lose appetite. But the birds drink more water. A green-yellow diarrhea is characteristic. Clinical signs of FT are indistinguishable from those of Pullorum disease. Birds less than 4 weeks of age have fecal pasting of the vent area. Onset of clinical signs in baby birds is 6 to 8 days of age. Mortality often reaches 40 to 50 percent. Surviving birds are stunted and unthrifty.

LESIONS AND DIAGNOSIS:

The lesions of FT are not diagnostic but do vary from those of pullorum or paratyphoid (other salmonella diseases). The liver and spleens are swollen and dark, have a metallic sheen and exhibit pin-point necrosis.The gall bladder becomes distended. Other typical signs of septicemia are pin-point hemorrhages in fat and muscle, muco-catarrhal enteritis, pasty vent areas of young birds and shriveled dis-colored yolks in ovary of hens. The birds are pale and anemic. The RBC count drops to 1.8 million cells/ml (normal count is 3.5 million cells/ml) and the WBC count increases to 24,000/ml (18,000 WBC is normal). Under certain circumstances, a presumptive diagnosis can be made on basis of history, signs, and lesions. Laboratory confirmation requires isolating and identifying the organism. The isolate must be differentiated, especially from pullorum and paratyphoid. The infec-tion is septicemic, so all organs and tissues can be sources for labora-tory isolation of the *S. gallinarum*.

TREATMENT AND CONTROL:

Fowl typhoid is a reportable disease; therefore, all confirmed out-breaks must be reported to the regulatory agencies. Fowl typhoid is a National Poultry Improvement Program (NPIP) disease controlled by eradication. Several sulfonamides, antibiotics, and antibacterials are effective in reducing mortality, but none will cure or eradicate the dis-ease from the flock. Medication will interfere with diagnosis. Eradica-tion of the disease is done under regulatory supervision which means that the entire flock must be destroyed. After flock depopulation, the equipment and premises must be cleaned and disinfected (C & D) to prevent carry-over of the disease. Even the C & D is done under close supervision. Environmental culturing to assure that the disease is eradicated will be performed.

Control then becomes an exercise of prevention. All producers are en-couraged to participate in the NPIP program which requires that ALL breeder-replacement flocks be pullorum-typhoid tested before bringing into production. The program is carried out by regulatory officials of each state; therefore, each producer needs to become acquainted with the program officials in his/her state. Testing procedures, but not test requirements, may vary from state to state.

The national program requires that 10 percent of each breeder flock (or 300 birds, whichever is greater) be tested. Some states accept the "whole-blood rapid plate test," and the flock owner or an agent of the flock owner may be trained and then certified as a tester of gamebird breeder birds. This program works well, and all gamebird producers should find out about the NPIP program in their states.

PREVENTION:

Fowl typhoid is handled only on eradication basis. After premise is released from quarantine, depopulation, and C& D, repopulation can begin but should include only birds from NPIP pullorum/typhoid-clean sources.

Gamebird production in future years must be as an NPIP participant whereby every breeder flock is pullorum/typhoid tested and found to be clean. In pullorum/typhoid-free states, certification is required for gamebirds and poultry for exhibition. Such birds must originate from NPIP participating flocks or be tested before admission to the show or competition. There is no public health hazard from this disease.

GOOSE SEPTICEMIA

Goose septicemia, a fowl cholera-like disease, is an acute contagious disease of geese and sometimes ducks and swans. It is caused by a bacterium and is characterized by septicemia, prostration, and death. The disease has been called goose influenza or fowl cholera, but in Europe it is referred to as goose septia. The causative agent is *Pasteurella septicaemia*, a gram negative encapsulated nonmotile nonspore-forming bipolar rod. Incubation of *P. septicaemia*, requires 3 to 9 days and its course is 2 weeks, or until flock is depopulated. The biochemical reactions are the same as those of *P. anatipestifer*. (*P. anatipestifer* infects ducks and turkeys.)

Some investigators believe the organisms are the same but the fact that duck and goose isolates show reduced virulence when inoculated into the opposite host from the isolation refutes that belief. All breeds and ages of geese are susceptible to the disease but it can be extremely serious in goslings and immature geese. The disease has been reported wherever geese are grown world wide, but is not serious in the USA because the bird numbers are small and most geese are grown in captivity.

TRANSMISSION AND CLINICAL SIGNS:

Goose septicemia is spread directly from bird to bird and from infected exudates in the feed, water, and premises to pen-mates. The disease is not spread in the egg; spread is entirely by direct contact or environmentally. Infection is shed to some level in the feces, so recovered birds are carriers. *P. multocida* is shed in the semen of infected turkeys; hence *P. septicaemiae* would probably be found in the semen of recovered ganders. As the name septicemia implies, clinical signs are rapid onset, coughing, sneezing, eye and nasal exudates. Infected birds are weak, become dehydrated, incoordinated, cyanotic, prostrate, and then die.

LESIONS AND DIAGNOSIS:

Inflammatory lesions prevail, including respiratory tissues, pericarditis, perihepatitis, caseous airsacculitis, peritonitis, swollen congested liver with irregular areas of necrosis (mottled). Spleen, kidneys, and reproductive organs are swollen, congested, and hemorrhagic. Fats are blood-tinged and have petechial hemorrhages. Lesions in liver and heart are suggestive of goose septicemia. A presumptive diagnosis can be based on the described history of the onset of the illness, clinical signs, and gross lesions. Laboratory confirmation requires the isolation and identification of the organism, *P. septicaemiae*. The isolate must be differentiated from *P. multocida*, *P. anatipestifer*, and *E. coli*.

TREATMENT AND CONTROL:

Sulfa drugs are generally effective. Sulfadimethoxine is the safer of the sulfonamides. Antibiotics, especially tetracycline, penicillin and novobiocin, will often be beneficial. The dosage of sulfa drugs is 1/2 oz in 1 gal drinking water for 3 days. Then reduce sulfa drug dosage to 1/2 oz in 2 gal drinking water.

In adult geese, penicillin is more effective when injected, but for goslings and juvenile birds it may be more effective administered [100 mg/gal] in the drinking water. Bacterins are recommended if available. For large flocks an autogenous bacterin should be made and used prophylactically for future hatches. Control requires treatment plus the correcting and upgrading of pen conditions. Continuous practice of good husbandry and hygiene will help to prevent a relapse of the disease.

PREVENTION:

Improved pen sanitation, flock husbandry, and strict biosecurity are absolute necessities if goose septicemia is to be prevented. New and healthy birds should be segregated from sick or exposed geese. Do not retain any goose from an outbreak flock. Isolate sick and recovered birds until marketed. It is important that you do not place new birds in exposed and infected pens. Therefore, thoroughly clean and disinfect pens, and leave them empty for at least 4 weeks.

Indoor dirt-floor pens should be treated with an application of formalin. Formalin is hazardous; therefore, the person applying the formalin should wear protective rubber wear and a respirator. Do not allow formalin to touch the skin. Start at one end of the building, go to other end, exit, and securely lock the doors to prevent access. Allow 24 to 48 hours before reentering, then open doors and windows to thoroughly ventilate the building, taking care that animals or people do not enter, endangering themselves and possibly recontaminating the premises. This treatment, properly executed, will eradicate the disease from the facility. There is no effective procedure for treating outdoor pens, but long periods of rest with tilling the soil and exposure to sunlight is helpful. For further assurance, vaccinate the next flock or two with an autogenous bacterin.

INFECTIOUS CORYZA

DEFINITION:

Infectious coryza (IC) is an infectious contagious respiratory bacterial disease of several avian species. At the onset, IC disease is acute to subacute, but it progresses to the chronic state as it works through the flock. Common names for the disease include roup, cold, and coryza. Chickens are the primary host of coryza, but pheasants, guinea fowl, and turkeys are also susceptible. In temperate climates, it is an important and serious disease of gamebirds and poultry, and it can be assumed that other gamebird species will become infected if they routinely commingle with chronically infected gamebirds or poultry flocks. Age-wise, coryza is a disease of juvenile and mature birds, or birds 14 weeks of age or older.

Coryza is characterized by nasal discharge, facial swelling, sneezing, labored breathing, and fetid odors of the exudates. It is a disease of the bird's upper respiratory tract (i.e., trachea, sinuses, and air passages of the head). Coryza occurs world wide, but in the United States is most usually found in small noncommercial menagerie or hobby-type flocks.

The IC causative agent is *Hemophilus paragallinarum*, a polar-staining, pleomorphic, nonmotile, gram-negative rod first described in 1920. There are three antigenic types (**A, B,** and **C**); they all share certain antigens. *H. paragallinarum* requires a special growth factor (the"*V*" factor) to grow in culture.

TRANSMISSION AND CLINICAL SIGNS:

Chronically ill birds are reservoirs of infection. Birds may appear healthy, yet be carriers. The disease is often unknowingly introduced into the flock when such carriers are added. Recovered birds remain carriers and shedders for life.

Transmission may be direct (i.e., by bird-to-bird contact), through inhalation of infectious aerosols coughed into the air, or by ingestion of contaminated feed and water. The organism can be transferred on contaminated clothing, equipment, and fomites.

Incubation requires 1 to 3 days. In the infected individual bird, the duration of the disease endures for 14 days, but IC's slow spread means that sick birds will be in the flock for several weeks. The presence of other respiratory infections, such as mycoplasma, will increase the duration and severity of illness and impact on flock growth and production.

Once a flock has been infected, it becomes and remains a constant threat to clean flocks. The clinical signs are those typical of an upper respiratory disease — sneezing, lacrimation, swollen face, and nasal exudates. The nasal exudates are clear, thick and sticky, and have a fetid or rotten odor. Sick birds will go off feed and water, become lethargic, sit humped, and have ruffled feathers and swollen faces. Some birds also have sinusitis. The facial swelling is primarily around the eye and does not always involve the infraorbital sinus.

Mortality can be as high as 50 percent but is usually no more than 20 percent. The course and mortality of the disease correlate with the virulence of the pathogen, effectiveness of treatment, and concomitant infections.

LESIONS AND DIAGNOSIS:

In its acute stage, the principal lesions of IC are swollen face, watery eyes, rhinitis, nasal exudates that become crusty on the beak around the nostrils and cheesy in the nostrils and sinuses. Eyelids stick together because of the exudate or of accumulation of cheesy exudate in the conjunctival sac. Early exudates are copious, grayish-yellowish, and thick and sticky. Other lesions include tracheitis, bronchitis, and (on occasion) airsacculitis. Exudates in the trachea produce rattling (rales).

A presumptive diagnosis can be rendered on the flock history, progress of the disease, and the lesions. The fetid odor of nasal exudates, when present, is diagnostic. Confirmation requires a laboratory diagnostic work-up with isolation and identification of the organism. The pathogen has a special growth-media requirement; therefore, the bacteriology laboratory must be alerted to the diagnostician's suspicion of infectious coryza (H. paragallinarum).

The organism can be found in a gram-stained smear of the nasal exudates. Cultures should be made from nostrils, eye, cleft, and trachea, plus from lungs or air sacs if lesions are present. A presumptive diagnosis of IC is adequate cause to begin treatment of the flock.

TREATMENT AND CONTROL:

Flock medication with a sulfonamide or other antibiotic is recommended. Various sulfonamides — sulfadimethoxine (SDM), (SQ), sulfamethazine (sulmet) are all effective; however, sulfadimethoxine is the safest and the one prescribed as treatment of choice. SQ and sulmet are more toxic and require intermittent administration. Therapy by way of the drinking water will give more immediate response and reduce the severity of the disease. Adding the sulfa or antibiotic to the feed extends the period of treatment and thereby provides better control.

For these reasons, a combined-treatment approach is advisable. Administer medication in the drinking water until medicated feed can be provided. Tetracycline, erythromycin, spectinomycin, and tylosin are beneficial, safe, and approved for use in poultry.

Control cannot be accomplished with drugs alone. Management is equally important. A bacterin that can be used in a control or eradication program is available. To be effective, the bacterin program requires multiple injections, and becomes costly and cumbersome for commercial flocks.

Control requires strict flock sanitation, biosecurity, preventive medication, clean and sanitary premises, and disease-free replacements.

PREVENTION:

Prevention requires eradication of the disease (depopulation if necessary), good husbandry, strict biosecurity, all in-all out management, raising your own breeder replacements, and no mixing of ages or species. Most outbreaks occur as a result of mixing flocks. If you do have an outbreak, segregate birds by age and species, burn dead birds, begin medication, and initiate eradication procedures. DO NOT SAVE RECOVERED BIRDS AS REPLACEMENT BREEDERS. Premises should be vacant for 30 to 60 days following cleaning and disinfecting. Obtain replacement breeders from an IC-clean source.

LISTERIOSIS

DEFINITION:

Listeriosis is an infectious disease of gamebirds and poultry caused by a bacterium. The disease is characterized by septicemia, encephalitis, and focal necrosis in abdominal organs. The causative agent is *Listeria monocytogenes*, a slender nonspore-forming, microaerophilic gram positive rod which grows well on blood agar and in chicken embryos. All age groups are susceptible but the disease is primarily diagnosed in young birds. All domestic breeds of birds including canaries are susceptible as are ruminant animals and people. This disease is ordinarily reported as a disease of ruminants but has been well documented in avian species. In fact, poultry has been implicated in cases of listeriosis diagnosed in people. Outbreaks in birds are sporadic, but losses up to 40 percent have been reported in broilers. Listeriosis occurs world wide but more frequently in temperate climates. Incubation requires from 36 hours to 52 days, and the course of the disease is from 1 to 14 days.

TRANSMISSION AND CLINICAL SIGNS:

Listeria infection follows inhalation or ingestion of *L. monocytogenes* or by entry of the organism through wounds. The disease does not spread bird to bird. The source of infection is an environment of manure, soil, and decaying organic materials. Listeria is a common isolate of poorly cured silage fed to ruminant animals. The organism can be isolated using regular laboratory media and procedures.

Listeriosis is more prevalent in birds on premises where the birds commingle or have regular contact with other types of animals, especially cattle and sheep. Birds can harbor the infection without being clinically ill. Clinical signs are vague but usually those as typically described for "sick birds" — lethargic, off feed, weak and death. Listeriosis occurs as an encephalitis in young birds which causes incoordination, paralysis, and torticollis (head over back).

LESIONS AND DIAGNOSIS:

Listeriosis causes a septicemic infection with focal necrosis of liver and myocardium, pericarditis, and encephalitis. Histologically lesions include microabscesses, gliosis, and perivascular cuffing in the medulla of the brain. In broiler outbreaks of the encephalitic form, the predominant symptom is torticollis; however, with the acute septicemic form, the liver abscesses, focal necrosis, and myocardial degeneration are common.

As symptoms may be vague or confusing, confirmation depends on isolation and identification of the organism. *L. monocytogenes* can be isolated from the blood or tissue lesions (especially brain tissue) of birds sick or dead from the disease. Culturing directly from the floor of the medulla (brain stem) will increase isolation success. Blood agar and other laboratory media can be used. In cases difficult to confirm, the listeria can be grown in chicken embryos.

Mice, rabbits, and guinea pigs are susceptible to experimental infection; therefore these animals can be used in agent-identification procedures. Serologically, *L. monocytogenes* has been divided into different serotypes based on flagellar (H) and somatic (O) antigens. Other immunological tests are available but offer varying degrees of success.

TREATMENT AND CONTROL:

L. monocytogenes is resistant to most of the commonly used antibiotics. High levels of tetracycline are usually prescribed. Newer antibiotics that become available may be worth using in treatment of Listeriosis. At the same time, any improvement in husbandry and flock hygiene will be helpful and is recommended. Prophylactic use of antibiotics may have benefits as a follow-up to initial treatment, as well as to unaffected flocks on the premises.

Since the disease does not respond well to medication, control must be achieved through management — i.e., effective biosecurity and superior husbandry. Early flock termination may prove to be the least costly method of control. Every biosecurity measure should be implemented to assure that the disease is contained in the affected flock or flocks.

PREVENTION:

Prevention of Listeriosis depends on finding and removing the source of infection. There is no reliable prophylactic procedure for this disease. Eradication of the infection is the only reliable and consistent method of prevention. Flock depopulation, pest and rodent control, careful C& D of the facilities followed by 30 days down time are the recommended disease-eradication procedures. Litter removed from bird pens should be composted, then applied and plowed under in cultivated fields located a considerable distance away from and inaccessible to poultry or livestock.

MYCOPLASMA GALLISEPTICUM

DEFINITION:

Mycoplasma gallisepticum (MG) is a contagious infectious disease of gamebirds and poultry of all ages. MG is caused by a bacterial-type organism and characterized by respiratory signs and sinusitis accompanied with a chronic prolonged course in the flock. Common names are MG, Mycoplasmosis, CRD (chickens), and infectious sinusitis (turkeys). MG is a pathogenic species within the genus *Mycoplasma* of microorganisms. The organism is sensitive to several antibiotics and easily destroyed by sanitizers, disinfectants, and sunlight. In the environment, MG will survive long periods in infected exudates, contaminated pens and litter, and in infected yolk materials as well. Most poultry diagnostic laboratories can culture MG from infected avian tissues and respiratory cultures. MG requires from 3 to 10 days for incubation, and its course is slow and long.

The list of susceptible avian hosts is long. MG is not contagious to other animals but birds of all ages, especially the young of pheasant, partridge, pea fowl, guinea fowl, pigeon, and quail are susceptible. MG occurs worldwide, wherever gamebirds and poultry are grown. It is not found in birds in the wild but is more directly linked to birds reared in captivity. Most noncommercial flocks, hobby and exhibition poultry flocks, pigeons, and many gamebird populations are infected with MG. Recovered birds remain carriers and shedders of the disease; consequently, once a flock is infected, it remains infected.

TRANSMISSION AND CLINICAL SIGNS:

M. gallisepticum is transmitted by several means. The disease spreads horizontally by contact from bird to bird, infected bird to litter, equipment, air-borne dust, and nasal droplets. MG is spread vertically from infected hen to chick by egg passage (trans-ovarian). MG can be isolated from the ovary and oviduct of hens as well as from semen of males in breeder flocks. Hatchlings from infected breeders are infected when hatched (vertical) and then infect penmates (horizontal). MG spreads to other pens and farms by visitors, farm workers, and caretakers on shoes, clothing, hands, crates, feed sacks, or equipment.

Nasal discharges and foamy-like secretions given off as aerosols from ill birds are infectious to susceptible contact birds. The disease spreads more rapidly within pens or areas of poor ventilation. Clinical signs develop slowly in the flock. Cold damp environment contributes to severity of the infection. Early signs are watery eyes, coughing, sneezing, rales, conjunctivitis, nasal discharge, and sinusitis (swelling of infraorbital sinus). These signs may not be noticed by caretakers because of the chronic nature of MG since birds in different stages of the disease are present within the flock. Partridge, turkeys, pea fowl, and some strains of pheasant will develop bilateral sinusitis. Recovered birds remain as carriers and shedders of MG.

LESIONS AND DIAGNOSIS:

MG-infected birds have upper-respiratory involvement and liberate muco-caseous exudates from the nostrils, sinuses, trachea, lungs, and air sacs (airsacculitis). Sinuses swell with liquid exudates that become caseous or cheesy. Eyes may matter shut. Birds lose weight, are un-thrifty, off feed, dehydrated, cyanotic, and have ruffled feathers. On necropsy, in addition to presence of exudates, the respiratory tissues and membranes are congested and dark. The abdominal organs will be congested, swollen, and dark. Lungs will contain microabscesses and the air sacs will be cloudy and contain a frothy to caseous exudate. A presumptive diagnosis can be rendered on basis of flock history, clinical signs, and gross lesions. Serological tests positive for MG and negative for other respiratory diseases are diagnostic. Confirmation requires the isolation and identification of the isolate. Flock medication should be initiated on the basis of presumptive diagnosis since laboratory confirmation takes 5 to 10 days. MG is sensitive to several antibiotics so positive response to medication is supportive evidence to the accuracy of the diagnosis. MG must be differentiated from other mycoplasma infections, Newcastle disease, and infectious coryza.

TREATMENT AND CONTROL:

MG is sensitive to Tylosin, erythromycin, Baytril (not yet approved in the USA), lincomycin, and spectinomycin. For Tylosin treatment of the flock, medication [2 g/gal] should be administered via water until infection is brought under control. Then medicate with Tylosin by feed [50 to 200 g/ton] for prolonged or continuous medication. Tylosin feed medication [50 to 100 g/ton] is recommended for infected breeder birds, especially if birds are of a rare breed. Flock medication is particularly effective for salvaging flocks for the season. It is unwise to save breeder replacements from MG-recovered flocks. Eradication is the more prudent approach for future years. MG is a NPIP-program disease; replacement birds should be from NPIP-member producers who have mycoplasma-free stock.

For rare bird lines, a program of individual bird treatment, vaccination, and antibiotic inoculation of eggs can be developed to preserve genetic lines. The program is labor intensive and expensive. When sufficient numbers of MG-free progeny are hatched and started, the infected breeder population should be terminated. Further control is dependent on effective management and flock biosecurity. For common commercial lines of gamebirds, purchasing MG-free replacements is far less costly and easier.

PREVENTION:

MG prevention is predicated on sole use of MG-free breeder stock, good husbandry, and an effective flock biosecurity program. MG is a NPIP control disease. It is recommended that all gamebird growers become NPIP participating members. The program requires annual blood testing of gamebird and poultry breeder flocks for MG, *M. synoviae, M. meleagridis*, Pullorum, and fowl typhoid. If the breeders are "clean" the progeny will be "clean." Growers should contact their state diagnostic laboratory for testing procedures. Breeder flocks found to be infected with MG should be slaughtered. It is less costly to act promptly and eradicate MG than it is to continue hatching from known infected breeders. This is true from one year to the next.

MYCOPLASMA MELEAGRIDIS

DEFINITION:

A widespread egg-transmitted infectious disease of turkeys and closely related species in which the primary lesion in progeny is airsacculitis. Common names include MM, N-strain, and H-strain. The causative organism, *Mycoplasma meleagridis* (MM), is related to but serologically distinct from other avian mycoplasmas. The organism is fastidious in its growth requirements but will grow in cell-free laboratory media that is enriched with serum. The incubation period is 5 to 10 days and the course of the disease is slow and long.

The primary host is the turkey, but peafowl, pigeon, and quail are susceptible. MM is susceptible to antibiotics and easily destroyed by environmental factors and disinfectants. MM has no public health significance. MM occurs world wide and the incidence of associated airsacculitis is high in progeny from infected breeders.

TRANSMISSION AND CLINICAL SIGNS:

MM tends to be a venereal disease of adult birds. The organism harbors in the reproductive tract of the breeder. Eggs become infected as they traverse down the oviduct. In the breeder male, the organism is retained in the genital phallus and adjacent tissues, contaminating the semen and the hen. In hens, the organism is retained in the bursa of Fabricius. The high rate of transmission is from infection of the reproductive tract. MM spreads from infected to susceptible pen-mates by respiratory aerosols or by people with contaminated hands during vent-sexing. Embryo infection reduces hatchability, progeny quality, and growth. Clinical signs in young birds are high mortality because of starve-outs. Birds are unthrifty, have respiratory illness, and stunted growth. Respiratory illness is the primary sign in juvenile to adult birds. Another sign is crippling resulting from skeletal deformity caused by osteomyelitis of the neck and legs. Adult birds may show no signs of the venereal or respiratory infections.

LESIONS AND DIAGNOSIS:

Infected, pipped, unhatched embryos and newly hatched birds have variable degrees of airsacculitis manifested by thickened membranes and yellow exudates. Hatchlings with crooked necks probably have infection in the cervical airsacs. Airsac lesions tend to recede as the bird matures. MM can cause a generalized skeletal disorder. In young birds, tracheitis and pneumonia may be present. Adult birds are usually free of lesions. Microscopic lesions in hens consist of lymphocytic foci in the oviduct. In infected birds, MM has been isolated from the respiratory tract, reproductive tracts, joints, and bursa of Fabricius. A presumptive diagnosis of MM can be based on typical history, clinical signs, and lesions. Confirmatory tests include positive serology, and isolation and identification of the agent. The disease must be differentiated from other mycoplasma, chlamydia, bacterial, and viral respiratory infections.

TREATMENT AND CONTROL:

Several antibiotics are effective against MM infections. Currently Tylosin and tetracycline are the drugs of choice. Other medications that offer benefits are Baytril (not FDA approved), LS 50, lincomycin, erythromycin, and spectinomycin. Follow label instructions to prepare correct dosage of the drug. Treatment programs should be used to salvage the present flock, but do not save birds for breeder replacement. However, no treatment is known to be effective against venereal MM so it must be eradicated to be controlled. Obtain replacement breeders from MM-free hatcheries. This can be accomplished by buying all stock, eggs or hatchlings, the succeeding year. Select future breeders from these birds. Mature birds specifically for breeding may be purchased. When the genetic line of current stock is not replaceable, then a special program of injecting each egg with an antibiotic preparation is required. Egg injection reduces hatchability but live hatchlings are free of mycoplasma. This strategy will preserve genetic lines, but is not recommended for commercial lines replaceable from other gamebird producers.

PREVENTION:

Maintain a mycoplasma-free breeder stock to prevent MM. The grower should establish a mycoplasma-monitoring program by blood testing breeders before production and periodically during the season. MM testing is a voluntary NPIP program. Examine and culture unhatched and pipped embryos for mycoplasma. Antibiotic injection is helpful for hatchlings from infected breeders or hatchlings scheduled for placement on infected premises. Tylosin in the drinking water 2 to 3 days per week for 3 weeks is an alternative to injecting each baby bird. Prevention is accomplished by starting with MM-free gamebirds and then monitoring breeder birds and unhatched progeny for early detection of outbreaks.

MYCOPLASMA SYNOVIAE

DEFINITION:

Mycoplasma synoviae is an infectious disease with worldwide distribution in chickens and turkeys, making it a threat to gamebirds. The disease is caused by a mycoplasma that is characterized by exudative tendonitis and bursitis. Common synonyms are MS, infectious synovitis, synovitis, and silent airsac. MS also produces a subclinical respiratory infection. The causative organism is *Mycoplasma synoviae*. There appears to be only one serotype.

The disease was first reported in 1954. The incubation period is 5 to 10 days and course of the disease is slow and prolonged. The organism, closely related to but serologically distinct from MG and MM, can be cultured on laboratory media or in embryonating chicken eggs. The organism has a predilection for synovial-lined structures, such as joints and tendon sheaths, but also localizes in the ovary of the hen. Most gamebird species are susceptible; therefore, they are at risk if housed near infected chickens or turkeys.

TRANSMISSION AND CLINICAL SIGNS:

MS is egg transmitted but at a much lower rate than other mycoplasmas. The respiratory form of the disease spreads from aerosols of infected birds to susceptible hatch-mates. MS can be contracted from an infected environment. One theory is biting insects such as lice, mites, ticks, and mosquitoes spread the disease from infected to susceptible birds. Caretakers can spread the disease from pen to pen on shoes, clothing, and hands.

Poor hygiene on the premises also perpetuates the disease. First clinical signs are lame birds with swollen hocks and foot pads filled with exudates. Affected birds are reluctant to move, have a stilted gait, lose weight, and develop breast blisters. Younger birds usually are more seriously affected. A few may exhibit signs of respiratory problems. Greenish diarrhea is common in dying birds. The respiratory form resembles MG. Morbidity is up to 15 percent with 10 percent mortality.

LESIONS AND DIAGNOSIS:

The most prevalent lesions are swollen and infected joints and breast blisters. The exudates of the joints and breast blisters are creamy-

spleen and fibrinous stringy exudates around the heart. Chronically infected birds become thin and dehydrated and develop a catarrhal enteritis and a greenish diarrhea. In the respiratory form, air sacs contain yellow caseous exudates.

A presumptive diagnosis can be based on clinical signs and lesions. Confirmation is dependent on positive serology and the isolation and identification of the agent M. synoviae and the absence of bacteria from joint exudates. Histologically, joints are infiltrated with heterophils and fibrin in the joint spaces, tendons, and synovial membranes. Articular cartilages of joints become thin and pitted. The walls of arteries of major organs are thickened and the thymus and bursa become atrophied. MS must be differentiated from MG, MM, and staphylococcosis.

TREATMENT AND CONTROL:

Several antibiotics, varying in effectiveness, are available. High levels of tetracycline are effective. Medication should be considered as a salvage effort as birds from infected flocks should not be kept for breeding. A treatment regimen where two antibiotics are administered simultaneously, one by feed and other by drinking water, will hasten control within the flock. Baytril, not presently FDA approved, is effective against all mycoplasma infections. Other effective antibiotics are tylosin, erythromycin, lincomycin, and spectinomycin. Recovery is slow for both the respiratory and the synovitis forms of the disease. To control MS, all birds must come from MS-free breeder flocks. Breeders should be tested and monitored for the disease throughout the season. Adult birds may be asymptomatic; however, infected breeders can be identified by serological tests. Flocks found to be infected should be terminated but can be salvaged for slaughter.

PREVENTION:

Eradication of MS is the only practical long-term control. Buy or hatch eggs from breeder flocks known to be M. synoviae free since it is possible to obtain gamebird chicks from MS-free sources. The breeder flock health program should include pre-season testing and monitoring for MS along with other NPIP diseases. All good husbandry practices and biosecurity are recommended to protect the health of all gamebird flocks.

NECROTOTIC ENTERITIS

DEFINITION:

Necrotic enteritis is an acute infectious catarrhal enteritis of gamebirds and poultry caused by a toxin-producing bacterium. The disease is characterized by necrosis of intestinal mucosa, rapid debilitation, and death. Synonyms are NE, enterotoxemia, and rot gut. The diseased is caused by *Clostridium perfringens*, a gram positive, anaerobic, spore-forming rod that grows in the intestinal tracts of birds and other animals.

Incubation requires 3 to 6 days and the course of the disease is 10 to 14 days. *C. perfringens* liberates several toxins. "**A**" and "**C**", both necrotoxins, are shown to be involved in birds. Necrotoxins cause tissue death on contact — in this case, the intestinal mucosa. The organism survives in the litter, especially in houses where litter has "built-up" or been used for several flocks. Young rapidly growing gamebirds, 4 to 16 weeks of age, are most susceptible. NE is frequently diagnosed in chukar and pheasants. A related disease, ulcerative enteritis or quail disease, commonly infects quail. Clostridia spores are commonly found in the soil, dust, and intestinal contents; therefore, the organism is present wherever gamebirds and poultry are grown. NE has been reported in most gamebird and poultry producing areas of the world. The disease is often masked by other more-recognizable diseases so may remain undiagnosed and unreported in an area for some time. Frequency and severity of necrotic enteritis are dependent on predisposing conditions.

TRANSMISSION AND CLINICAL SIGNS:

Necrotic enteritis is a soil-borne disease. The bacterium is ingested from soil, dust, or fecal matter. Once ingested, the organism grows within the intestine and there secretes the necrotoxins that damage the mucus membrane for which the disease is named — necrotic enteritis.

The disease most commonly occurs in flocks kept in high-density and crowded environments. Once present, it progresses rapidly throughout the flock. The great quantity of bacteria shed in the feces enhances spread by fecal-oral route. Feces of infected birds are a fetid brownish liquid. Birds are depressed, lose appetite, and have diarrhea with dark feces that may be tinged with blood.

Clinical features progress rapidly as death occurs within a few hours. The disease persists in untreated flocks for approximately 10 days.

Mortality ranges from 2 to 50 percent. Chronically affected birds become emaciated and have necrotic and hemorrhagic lesions on the feet. The disease is complicated by other diseases of gamebirds, especially histomoniasis, ulcerative enteritis, coccidiosis, and capillariasis.

LESIONS AND DIAGNOSIS:

The infected bird is thin and dehydrated with brown diarrhea. The breast muscle is dark and cyanotic; liver is swollen and congested; intestine is ballooned, friable, and filled with fetid brown liquid contents; and the intestinal mucosa is covered with a brownish necrotic diphtheritic membrane. Large numbers of short thick gram positive rods can be seen on stained smears of mucosal scrapings. In advanced cases, the swollen liver develops circumscribed necrotic areas and bone marrow is pale. Histopathological lesions confirm a coagulative necrosis of the mucus membrane and masses of clostridial-like bacteria in the fibro-necrotic debris. Diagnosis is confirmed by culturing anaerobically C. perfringens from the intestinal contents.

All toxigenic strains of the bacterium are identical. Differentiation requires toxin-neutralization tests to determine the presence of specific toxins. A presumptive diagnosis can be based on history, clinical signs, and lesions but confirmation requires isolation and identification of the C. perfringens. NE is often complicated by coccidiosis in younger infected flocks. It is important to recognize the severity of the coccidiosis whether it is primary or secondary in the outbreak. Unless coccidiosis is a primary factor, then attention and treatment should be focused on NE.

TREATMENT AND CONTROL:

Most clostridia are sensitive to many antibiotics, including bacitracin, lincomycin, neomycin, streptomycin, and tetracycline. A successful approach for control of outbreaks is one antibiotic in the feed and another in the drinking water for several days or until mortality stops. Then discontinue the water medication but continue the feed medication up to 14 days. In the meantime, upgrade sanitation and hygiene within the pen. Litter should be changed if there is manure build-up. Also, initiate treatment for concomitant infections as coccidiosis and histomoniasis.

On-wire rearing often is recommended especially for chukar and quail to prevent clostridia bacteria that are harbored in the feces and environment. Control relies more on improved management, hygiene and early detection of infection. Environmentally induced diseases can occur in birds on wire but keeping birds from contact with their feces prevents heavy exposure to the pathogens. Preventive medications are commonly used to control clostridial disease in highly susceptible bird species. For example, bacitracin [100 g/ton] is often used on a continuous basis in quail feeds Other antibiotics can be used but the drug dosage varies with each antibiotic. Follow prescribed levels for each drug used.

PREVENTION:

Prevention should be directed toward husbandry and management. The grower should become acquainted with the susceptibility of specific diseases for the respective gamebird species being grown. A management strategy, such as on-wire rearing, e.g., is recommended for chukar and quail. By adapting the husbandry specifically to minimize inherent gamebird species problems, every flock should be more successful. To break the cycle of disease, the flock may need to be depopulated followed with comprehensive cleaning and disinfecting. All predisposing factors should be reviewed and corrections made before repopulating. Excellent husbandry and biosecurity should be daily practice.

OMPHALITIS

DEFINITION:

Omphalitis, a nonspecific infection of the navel and yolk sac, is most frequently seen in new hatchlings. This disease occurs worldwide and is associated with contamination of the incubating equipment and/or the setting of dirty or cracked eggs. Since the problem is directly related to the incubator and hatching-egg sanitation, eggs that explode during incubation contaminate all eggs in the machine. The condition is also called "navel ill," "mushy chick," and "early chick" disease.

Omphalitis is characterized by unhealed navels and abdominal edema. It is caused primarily by coliform bacteria. Other factors, such as excessive incubator humidity, and chilling or overheating newly hatched birds contribute to the severity of the problem. Hatching eggs with poor shell quality produces a higher incidence of omphalitis. The incubation period is 8 to 16 hours and course of the disease is 6 to 7 days. All avian species are susceptible. Omphalitis is more prevalent in gallinaceous birds than in waterfowl species.

TRANSMISSION AND CLINICAL SIGNS:

Infection occurs at the time of hatching, before chicks with unhealed navels are removed from the incubator. Opportunistic bacteria (coliforms) are often recovered from infected birds. Proteolytic anaerobes are also prevalent in serious outbreaks. Losses may be increased by chilling or over-heating hatchlings during shipment.

Omphalitis does not spread from chick to chick. It is contracted within the environment from dirty trays, shells, or shipping containers. The affected hatchling appears normal the first few days. As infection becomes septicemic and toxic, the chick becomes weak and unthrifty with enlarged "mushy" (soft edematous) abdomen, moist inflamed navel, and pasted vent.

The birds are feverish so they huddle and make sounds of discomfort. Most infected birds die within the first week; hence the name "early chick" disease. Incidence and losses vary from hatch to hatch, depending on incubator sanitation and breeder-flock source (quality of egg shells). Egg shell quality deteriorates as breeders get older. Mortalities of 10 to 15 percent have been reported but expected range is 1 to 3 percent. Mortality equals morbidity because infected chicks die the first week.

LESIONS AND DIAGNOSIS:

The naval is inflamed and edematous with the possibility of a scab formation. The yolk sac remains large with a liquefied yolk. The bird has peritonitis with a rotten odor and fibrinous exudates that adhere to the navel. Other lesions are edema of the skin of abdomen, septicemia, and dehydration. Mortality may begin at hatching and continue throughout the first week of brooding. Persistent unabsorbed infected yolks usually cause stunting and general unthriftiness. A tentative diagnosis can be based on the presence of lesions at the time of necropsy. Yolk sac material, peritonitis, edema, and exudates should be cultured.

Omphalitis is always bacterial. Viral and other pathogenic agents are not directly involved. Bacterial isolation and identification are needed to determine source and probability of an ongoing problem. Omphalitis occurs industry-wide, but outbreaks are problems for the farm or company, and not for the industry.

TREATMENT AND CONTROL:

There is no effective treatment for Omphalitis. Most affected hatchlings die within the first few days. When mortality exceeds 3 percent, the operation should be investigated for egg shell quality, egg handling-sanitation, incubation-hatching procedures, machine sanitation, and other possible contributing sources such as personnel, ventilation, etc. Treatment and control efforts must be directed toward the prevention of omphalitis in future hatches. Give particular attention to egg washing procedures. Critical to egg sanitation is time, temperature, frequency of water changes, and concentration of the sanitizer. Eggs with sound shells should be saved but dirty eggs should be washed before sanitized. The rinse water following sanitizing should be warmer but should not exceed 140° Fahrenheit (60°C). The incubator should be cleaned and fumigated or heat fogged before the first setting of the season and between subsequent settings. Likewise, the hatching machinery should be cleaned and sanitized after each hatch. Do not mix settings in the hatcher. Incubator-hatcher rooms should be warm and have adequate safe ventilation, proper humidity, and be heat fogged at least weekly. As hatchery maintenance improves, the incidence of omphalitis will decrease.

PREVENTION:

Prevention of Omphalitis requires thorough sanitation control. In other words, control is by prevention through effective hatchery sanitation, surveillance of the breeder flock , and proper handling of eggs. Investigative procedures should include pullorum and paratyphoid status of breeder flocks, checking the cleanliness, temperature, and humidity of egg-holding rooms, sanitation of delivery trucks, used chick boxes, and brooding facilities. Only after correcting problems inherent at all points can the producer be assured that Omphalitis can be prevented.

PARATYPHOID

DEFINITION:

Paratyphoid is an acute to chronic febrile disease caused by salmonellae bacteria, and characterized by diarrhea, septicemia, and death in gamebirds and poultry as well as many other birds and mammals. The disease is often referred to as "salmonellosis and PT." The pathogens constitute a large genus of bacteria called salmonella. The genus is considered to have 2000 serotypes, 20 to 40 of which are more pathogenic to gamebirds and poultry. Each serotype has the capability to cross-infect other birds, animals, and people.

S. typhimurium alone accounts for approximately one-half the outbreaks in birds. The bacterium can be distinguished from pullorum and fowl typhoid by cell-structure and biochemical properties. PT infections are among the bacterial diseases most important to the hatching industry. They result in high death losses in all types of young birds. One estimate puts PT losses in USA at $77 million per year. The public health significance warrants serious attention. Severe illness occurs in young birds, especially those from 7 to 35 days of age. Mortality is generally in the range of 5 to 20 percent. PT infections exist in all parts of the world. Certain serotypes may predominate within a region. Most outbreaks in the USA can be attributed to one or more of 20 serotypes.

TRANSMISSION AND CLINICAL SIGNS:

The fact that salmonellae are able to survive and multiply in the environment is an important factor in their transmission. Litter, feedstuffs, dust, feces, hatchery fluff, soil, water, and vegetation all serve as reservoirs for salmonellae. In gamebirds and poultry, transmission primarily occurs from infected breeders by contamination of the egg shell, breakdown of hatchery sanitation, and lateral spread from infected birds in brooding and growing pens. In adult birds, the infection localizes in the intestine and gall bladder. Eggs become contaminated as they are laid. Hatchlings become infected from contact with infected egg shells at hatching.

Further spread occurs in chick boxes and brooder houses with exposure by ingestion of the infectious materials. Rodents, pets, and flies are primary vectors to the spread and maintainence of paratyphoid within the building as well as spread to adjacent facilities. A breakdown of husbandry becomes a mechanism of disease transfer within and among buildings and flocks. Clinical signs appear and the most severe stage occurs when the birds are between 7 and 28 days of age. Early signs would be depression, fever, and diarrhea, followed by dehydration and pasting of the vent areas. Birds go off-feed, have increased thirst, and develop swollen joints.

Clinical signs are not diagnostic because the same signs are common to a variety of enteric diseases. Morbidity is high to 28 days and mortality varies with the virulence of the pathogen in the outbreak. Outbreaks increase in severity as they spread to successive broods.

LESIONS AND DIAGNOSIS:

In acute outbreaks in young birds, gross lesions may be absent. Swollen liver, septicemia, emaciation, dehydration, retained yolk sac, enteritis with cheesy core, necrotic foci on organs, engorged blood vessels, and pale-yellow mottled liver are the predominant lesions. Less frequently found lesions are blindness, joint infections, and swollen eyelids, the latter two being more common in pigeons. Birds become stunted and flock will lack size uniformity. Mature birds show only enteritis and diarrhea.

A presumptive diagnosis can be based on history of onset, clinical signs, and lesions. The causative organism must be isolated and identified to confirm the disease as PT. Laboratory cultures should be taken from several organs. Serological tests should be done for pullorum and *S. typhimurium*; then the isolate should be serotyped. Paratyphoid should be differentiated from pullorum, fowl typhoid, colibacillosis, and other coliform enteritic infections. A complete laboratory diagnosis requires approximately 5 days. All salmonella infections must be reported to the state regulatory agency. A culture of the isolate should be submitted by diagnostic laboratory to the National Animal Disease Center for serotype confirmation.

TREATMENT AND CONTROL:

Recovered birds remain carriers. It is therefore recommended that a producer obtain breeder replacements from flocks free of PT. Treatment suppresses, but does not eliminate, infections. PT organisms are sensitive to antibiotics and sulfa drugs. The more effective ones are gentamicin, neomycin, spectinomycin, tetracycline, and sulfas. Sulfadimethoxine (SDM) is less toxic than other sulfa drugs.

Other sulfas are effective but must be used more judiciously. Gentamicin is effective but approved only for injection of poults at one day of age. A producer must be acquainted with the proper use of any medication, as most medicines are toxic at high dosages or when improperly used.

Remove and properly dispose of sick and dying or dead birds. Disposal should be by burning or deep burial. Control requires a coordinated approach, using the combination of i) medication, ii) adjust room temperature to comfort of birds, iii) supply fresh feed and water to encourage eating and drinking, iv) keep dead birds picked up and disposed of, v) maintain good sanitation and biosecurity, and vi) replace breeder stock from disease-free flocks (RECOVERED BIRDS REMAIN CARRIERS FOR LIFE).

PREVENTION:

Use only salmonella-free breeders. Raise new broods in the all-in, all-out systems. Before onset of production, breeders should be pullorum tested and monitored for PT by fecal and environmental culturing. Strict attention should be focused on hatchery and flock sanitation. Adult intestinal carriers are the main source of PT in new production seasons. Direct preventative measures are:

1. Sanitize the hatchery
2. Set only clean sanitized or fumigated eggs
3. Do not mix eggs from different flocks
4. Do not mix birds of different ages
5. Do not mix birds of different species.

PASTEURELLA ANATIPESTIFER

DEFINITION:

Pasteurella (Riemerella) anatipestifer (PA) is an acute to chronic, widely distributed contagious disease of ducks, turkeys, pheasants, and chickens. The disease is characterized by fibrinous pericarditis, perihepatitis, and paralysis. PA synonyms include new duck disease, duck septicemia, anatipestifer syndrome, and infectious serositis.

The causal agent, *Pasteurella (to* be renamed *Riemerella) anatipestifer,* is a gram negative, nonmotile, nonspore-forming rod that occurs singly, in pairs, and occasionally as filaments. Many cells stain bipolar with Wright's stain. The organism contains a capsule and is difficult to grow on laboratory media. Eight serotypes have been reported.

The organism can be isolated from heart blood, brain, air sacs, and liver of infected birds. PA was first described on Long Island, NY in 1932 in ducks reared in captivity. Once considered a disease of domestic ducklings 1 to 8 weeks of age, PA now shows ability to cause serious disease in other species, especially turkeys. Incubation requires 3 to 9 days and the course of the disease is 3 to 5 weeks. The disease occurs worldwide, is problematic in countries with intensive duck production, and persists in the environment. PA accounts for major economic losses to the duck industry due to high mortality, weight loss, and condemnations.

TRANSMISSION AND CLINICAL SIGNS:

The transmission of PA is by ingestion of organisms via contaminated feed, water, or litter. Further spread is by dust inhalation and wounds, e.g., toenail scratches. The organism can be spread from pen to pen by caretakers and others on contaminated shoes, clothing, and hands. Morbidity and mortality are always most severe in unsanitary pens.

The disease begins with a sudden onset within the flock and becomes more acute in new birds added to the brood. Early signs are respiratory — coughing, sneezing, ocular and nasal discharges; dehydration and greenish diarrhea; incoordination, weakness, and tremors of head and neck; coma; and death. Some of the birds lie on their backs and paddle. Mortality ranges from 5 to 75 percent. Condemnations of 3 to 13 percent has been reported. Stunting follows recovery from the acute phase of PA. A few ducks within the acutely ill flock may exhibit additional neurological signs. The virulence of the responsible pathogen accounts for the variations in severity of signs, lesions, and total mortality.

LESIONS AND DIAGNOSIS:

The most obvious lesion in ducks is the fibrinous exudate over the pericardial sac and over the surface of the liver. Lesions typical in birds of any species include fibrinous airsacculitis, caseous salpingitis in the female, arthritis, cyanosis, caseous pneumonia, and fibrinous meningitis. During the acute phase, septicemia with vascular engorgement, swollen liver, and other abnormal organs are predominant lesions. Chronic localized infections occur in skin and joints. Skin lesions are in the form of necrotic dermatitis of lower back or around vent. Yellowish exudate develops between the skin and fat layers.

The initial diagnosis is based on history, signs, and lesions. PA must be confirmed by isolation and identification of organism.

Suitable tissues for cultures are heart blood, liver, brain, air sacs, bone marrow, lung, exudates, and sinuses. Specimens should be taken aseptically. Laboratory medias include blood agar and trypticase soy agar, then incubation in reduced-oxygen atmosphere at 37°C for 24 to 72 hours. The isolate must be differentiated from other pasteurella diseases (fowl cholera and goose septicemia), colibacillosis, and other coliform septicemias. July and August are typical months of colibacillosis outbreaks. These diseases flourish in unsanitary pens and adverse environments.

TREATMENT AND CONTROL:

Antibiotics and sulfa drugs are effective in stopping mortality. Initial medication should be with sulfa drugs. Sulfadimethoxine (SDM) is a newer, safer, recommended sulfa. It can be administered in the feed or drinking water. Medication by drinking water gives quicker results. If the feed route is selected, provide the medication in the drinking water as well, but keep in mind that medication by the two routes MAY OVERLAP FOR NO MORE THAN ONE DAY. SDM can be administered for 7 days continuously whereas other sulfas require an interrupted medication sequence.

Antibiotics are beneficial after flock mortality is under control. Tetracycline is more effective than other antibiotics but streptomycin, erythromycin, novobiocin, and gentamicin are somewhat beneficial. Bacterins and live vaccines are commercially available, but should be used as part of a treatment and control program. SPECIAL NOTE: DO NOT USE THE LIVE VACCINE IN REPLACEMENT BIRDS.

PA control has to be accomplished through management, since treatment (dependent upon the severity of the outbreak) is expensive. Eradication of the disease, including depopulation of the current infected flock, is essential for long-term control on the premises.

DO NOT CARRY RECOVERED BIRDS OVER TO THE FOLLOWING YEAR. When a building becomes empty for the season, it should be thoroughly cleaned and disinfected, followed by fumigation if fumigate materials are obtainable, or by heat fogging. After fumigation, close and lock the building for several weeks.

PREVENTION:

Careful management is important for the prevention of PA but rigid sanitation and depopulation is required for eradication. Prevention requires immediate upgrading of sanitation, incineration of dead birds and isolation of outbreak flock to stop on-farm spread. Thoroughly clean and disinfect all facilities after infected flock is depopulated. Leave the disinfected pens empty for 4 weeks. A bacterin (killed vaccine) would be safe and recommended for the first flock following the disease eradication procedures. Successful prevention is by good management, good husbandry, and biosecurity.

PULLORUM DISEASE

DEFINITION:

Pullorum disease is an acute to chronic, contagious, infectious egg-transmitted disease whose natural hosts are domestic poultry, all gamebird species, song birds, hawks, parrots, and ratites. Many rodents and small-mammal species are susceptible to, but not seriously affected by, the disease. People are not susceptible. Synonyms include PD, bacillary white diarrhea, or BWD. The disease is caused by a bacterium, *Salmonella pullorum*, a gram negative nonmotile bacillus. The incubation period is 4 to 5 days, but the organism will survive up to a year in infected empty buildings. The course of the disease is 3 to 5 weeks.

Salmonella pullorum is resistant to cold, sunlight, dryness, and disinfectants. Pullorum disease is characterized by white diarrhea, high mortality in young birds, focal necrosis in organs, and asymptomatic adult carriers. PD occurs all over the world wherever poultry is grown, but infection in domestic poultry is rare. The disease has virtually been eradicated from commercial poultry but remains endemic in a few noncommercial and hobby flocks.

Young birds 7 to 28 days of age are the most susceptible. PD becomes inapparent in adult birds that are still carriers and shedders. In 1935 the National Poultry Improvement Program (NPIP) was organized after it was discovered that infected birds could be identified by blood tests. NPIP classified PD as a "controlled" disease. For a state to be classified as Pullorum-free, all breeding stock of gamebirds, waterfowl, exhibition, and commercial poultry must be tested. Pullorum test results must be negative before birds can be brought into production of hatching eggs. Positive blood tests must be reported to the State Veterinarian's Office. In accordance with the national plan, infected flocks are terminated. Premises are cleaned and disinfected under the supervision of regulatory inspectors.

TRANSMISSION AND CLINICAL SIGNS:

S. pullorum is spread primarily through eggs from infected hens to progeny. When a disease is spread from the hen to the chick, it is called a vertical transmission. Once introduced, PD spreads by various additional means, including contamination of incubators, hatchers, chick boxes, and infected houses, equipment, and feed. Carrier-shedder birds remain a threat to Pullorum-free status.

The bacterium localizes in the ovary and gall bladder of the hen and is shed in egg and feces. Infection occurs from ingestion of infected feces or feed or water. Spread among young birds is rapid. Early signs of the disease include small, weak, and dying hatchlings. Onset of mortality occurs about 8 days post-hatch. Morbidity and mortality increase daily.

Individual clinical signs are small stunted birds, loss of appetite, feverish birds, huddling birds, diarrhea, dehydration, weakness, pasted vent, gasping, and chalk-white feces sometimes stained with bile (green). By the fourth week, the flock appears to have three or four ages of birds. In the presence of other forms of stress — such as shipping, chilling, overheating, or poor sanitation — mortality can reach 100 percent.

It is also possible to have almost no mortality, in which case the disease might go unrecognized. PD today is usually introduceded by the purchase of infected stock or eggs. PD can be widely disseminated from hatcheries that do custom hatching of a menagerie of species. Such a hatchery must be shut down, cleaned, and disinfected to eradicate PD.

LESIONS AND DIAGNOSIS:

Deaths during an acute phase may not produce typical lesions but there will be a generalized septicemia. Lesions in young birds include unabsorbed yolk sacs; swollen liver and spleen; grayish nodules in the lungs, heart, and gizzard muscle; firm cheesy material in the ceca; raised proliferative lesions in the mucosa of the opened intestine; and white diarrhea with pasted vents.

Adult birds show regression of the ovary with shrunken greenish ova or testes, pericarditis, and focal necrosis of the liver. Many adult carrier birds will have no gross lesions. Later in the course of the disease a few birds may have swollen joints. However, joint lesions are more common in infected pigeons. Nodules and cecal cores may be found in birds that die 3 to 4 weeks into the course of the disease. History, symptoms, and lesions offer a probable diagnosis especially if birds are serologically positive on the blood test. Since gross lesions are similar to paratyphoid and other septicemic diseases, confirmatory tests are essential. Diagnosis is confirmed by isolation and identification of the pathogen.

Incorrect diagnosis of pullorum would create many problems for the flock owner and regulatory officials. Federal law requires that pullorum isolates be sent to the National Veterinary Services Laboratory for final definitive identification. When positive, a series of protective actions is initiated. The appropriate Federal and State regulatory agencies are notified. The flock is visited and quarantined. Arrangements are made for premise depopulation and disinfection. Under Federal-State supervision, birds are euthanatized, burned or buried, and the premises cleaned and disinfected. When the area is judged to be free of pullorum and typhoid, the quarantine is lifted and the producer is free to re-establish the production of gamebirds and/or poultry.

TREATMENT AND CONTROL:

There is no cure for pullorum disease. *S. pullorum* is sensitive to antibiotics and sulfas; therefore, with permission from the regulatory agencies, drugs may be used in order to salvage a flock for slaughter. Medication is known to induce the carrier state in recovered birds and would therefore serve to perpetuate PD.

Control of PD is based on each gamebird breeder becoming a member of NPIP. The program requires that all breeder flocks be tested and results be negative for PD. These blood tests should be conducted before the onset of production each year. The control of PD is critical to the health and well being of the gamebird and poultry industries. There are five officially approved pullorum tests. One is the whole-blood plate-agglutination test; it can be done by the producer on the premises.

All gamebird growers are encouraged to become NPIP participants. Most states have programs for training and certifying producers or producers' representatives as pullorum testers. The NPIP requires that 10 percent or 300 birds, normal male/female ratio, be tested and found negative before onset of production. Federal flock test forms V S 9-2 are then completed and sent to the state's official NPIP representative who reports this information to the national headquarters at Conyers, GA. The owner is assigned a NPIP flock number which identifies that flock as pullorum-free. This flock number should be used on all official reports, shipping forms, and advertising. Once a flock is classified as pullorum-free, never add new birds to the resident flock unless the new birds are also from a pullorum-free and NPIP member flock.

All birds of unknown pullorum status should be tested and negative before being released into the flock. Contact your state's NPIP representative for details, benefits, and requirements of this program.

PREVENTION:

Pullorum disease is so invasive that eradication is the only prudent method of control and prevention. No one would knowingly buy gamebirds infected with Pullorum. NPIP participation is the only wise choice for preventing PD.

Flocks not PD-free are totally eradicated by state officials, with the grower and Federal officials assisting. The NPIP is a cooperative program; its partners are the Federal and State regulatory agencies and the producer. Prevention is accomplished only by using known pullorum-free breeders. Only breeders need to be tested. If the parent birds are pullorum-free, so will be the progeny.

On any official test, reactor birds are submitted to the official state diagnostic laboratory for retest. Cultures from the organs are used for isolation of *S. pullorum*. If Pullorum is not isolated, the flock retains its Pullorum-free status.

SPIROCHETOSIS

DEFINITION:

Spirochetosis is a naturally occurring infectious septicemic vector-borne disease of most gamebird species, domestic fowl, waterfowl, canaries, and other birds. The disease is characterized by marked illness, depression, cyanosis, diarrhea, weakness, and paralysis. Spirochetosis is also called *Spirochetosis anserina, S. gallinarum, S. anatis,* and *Treponema serenum. Borrelia anserina,* a spirochete bacterium with five to eight spirals and up to 30 μ in length is the cause of the disease. *B. anserina* does not have the terminal hooks as seen in the leptospira bacteria and can be stained with aniline dyes and Romanowski stains.

The organism is motile and helical in shape. Spirochetes can be identified in wet smears of blood or tissues examined by darkfield microscopy. *B. anserina* can be propagated in special laboratory media but loses its virulence after 12 passages. For maintenance, *B. anserina* is serially passed in infected ticks or propagated in avian embryos by yolk-sac inoculation. The incubation period is 3 to 5 days and the course (viremic) is 3 to 5 weeks. Birds of all ages are susceptible, but chicks younger than 3 weeks are the most susceptible. A spirochetemia in infected chick lasts 2 to 3 weeks, compared with the 3 to 5 days that is usual in older birds. The organism is not resistant outside the host. The fowl tick serves as the reservoir. Spirochetes survive in carriers up to 31 days. Cultures can be maintained for extended periods at -70°C. Spirochetosis occurs world-wide but most frequently in tropical and subtropical climates. It has been recognized in Arizona, California, New Mexico, and Texas. The disease is important in countries where it is enzootic. In the southwest USA, there is a potential for spread with the prevalence of the tick vector, *Argas persicus.*

TRANSMISSION AND CLINICAL SIGNS:

Borrelia anserina is transmitted by blood-feeding vectors, especially *Argas persicus* (the fowl tick), culex mosquitoes, and avian mites. The organism can be transmitted by any direct transfer of infected blood, tissue, or excreta while cannibalizing moribund birds; or by ingesting blood, infected ticks, or feces or indirectly by eating contaminated feed or water. The primary vector, *Argas persicus,* remains infected as long as 430 days. The infected tick also passes the spirochete to its progeny. *B. anserina* is incapable of surviving in the bird or environment, therefore the *Argas persicus* tick becomes the principal reservoir for its perpetuation. Seven days after the tick feeds on a source of *B. anserina*, the spirochete reaches its salivary glands, ready to move on into the birds upon which the tick feeds. The tick's gonads serve as a source for the perpetuation of the disease through the tick progeny. Ticks become infective within 7 days after biting the host (an infected bird) and remain infected for 15 to 18 months. Larval ticks remain attached to the bird to feed for 4 to 5 days. Tick activity increases in warming temperatures, 35°C (93°F), and higher humidities. Recovered birds are not carriers. The organism dies when it leaves the bird.

Birds with *B. anserina* are visibly sick. They huddle, have droopy cyanotic heads and ruffled feathers, have diarrhea, and are anorexic. Birds are feverish with body temperatures of 111°F (normal is 105 to 107°F). Feces are liquid and green with excessive urates. Birds become weak, incoordinated, paralytic, anemic, comatose, and die. Recovering birds are thin and exhibit transient weakness or paralysis of the wings. Clinical signs may be absent in birds infected with strains low in pathogenicity.

LESIONS AND DIAGNOSIS:

The primary lesion is enlargement and mottling of the spleen. The liver is moderately swollen with multiple small hemorrhages and infarcts or necrotic foci. The kidney and heart are enlarged and pale. Intestines show bile staining with a presence of mucoid enteritis. Hemorrhage is present at the proventriculus-ventriculus junction. Occasionally a mild fibrinous pericarditis may be present. Other serous membranes are clear and not involved. Diagnosis relies on demonstrating the spirochete.

The disease should be suspected when immature fowl ticks are found on sick birds. Adult and nymph *Argas persicus* are nocturnal feeders and are not found on birds in daytime. The organism can be demonstrated on Giemsa-stained smears or by dark field or phase-contrast microscopy. Spirochetes may be concentrated in the white blood cell layer of a centrifuged heparinized blood sample. The test is useful for birds with low spirochete counts. The organism may be present but difficult to demonstrate in late stages of the disease.

The confirmatory test is inoculation of 6-day-old chicken embryos. Alternatively, chicks or poults can be inoculated with suspect serum or tissue suspensions, then blood smears examined daily for 3 to 5 days. The fluorescent antibody (FA) test is reliable on blood and tissue specimens. Agar gel precipitin test on serum will detect antibodies. Several effective serological tests have been developed, but due to the low incidence, many laboratories do not maintain the needed reagents. During outbreaks, regional laboratories acquire the materials needed for a rapid and accurate diagnosis.

TREATMENT AND CONTROL:

All cases should be reported promptly to regulatory authorities. In countries where Spirochetosis is endemic, a variety of drugs and antibiotics, including penicillin, is effective. At one time, a number of arsenicals were used in the treatment of Spirochetosis, but today, antibiotics are safer as well as more effective. Beneficial antibiotics are penicillin, chloramphenicol, kanamycin, streptomycin, tylosin, and tetracycline. Producers are advised to use only drugs that have been FDA approved for poultry and to abide by the proper withdrawal times before gamebirds are slaughtered or released.

Control is best accomplished by prevention, e.g., avoiding introduction of tick-infested birds into the flock and eradicating the fowl tick. Tick eradication may require the burning of all wooden buildings and destroying all infected flocks. Larval ticks can be controlled by dipping birds in 0.5% malathion. High-pressure spraying of building with a 3% malathion solution gives some measure of tick control. Control of Spirochetosis is dependent on effective elimination of the fowl tick — usually requiring radical and costly procedures.

PREVENTION:

Prevention requires effective control of the transmitting vectors, i.e., the fowl tick (*Argas persicus*), fowl mites, and culex mosquitoes. Only the tick is capable of harboring *B. anserina* (spirochetes) for long periods. Ticks remain infected 16 to 18 months. The primary control effort is directed toward the tick. In nonendemic areas, producers are urged not to bring in adult birds from endemic areas, but instead to bring in day-old hatchlings or fertile eggs for on-premise hatching.

Avoid introduction of adult birds that might be tick-infested or infected with *B. anserina*. Bacterins and vaccines manufactured in other countries have not been approved for use in the US. Apparently these products are useful, but costly (e.g., they require repeated vaccinations). Currently, Spirochetosis is not a known problem in the USA, but it has been reported in some southwestern states. Conditions in our southern climates favor the vectors. This is why the introduction of the infection into the vector population would trigger an ongoing gamebird problem. **Be aware of** and **avoid** imported gamebirds.

STAPHYLOCOCCOSIS

DEFINITION:

Staphylococcosis is an infectious bacterial disease of gamebirds and all classes of poultry with worldwide distribution. Birds less than 6 weeks of age are very susceptible; however, severe outbreaks in commercial turkeys of near market age have been reported. It is often called Staph infection, septicemia, arthritis, and bumblefoot. The incubation period for Staphylococcosis is 1 to 3 days and the course of the disease is 3 to 5 weeks.

The disease is characterized by septicemia in the acute phase and purulent synovitis manifested as bumblefoot, arthritis, or both, in the chronic phase. The causative agent is *Staphylococcus aureus*, a gram positive cocci that forms grape-like clusters on stained smears. It is an opportunistic pathogen; and therefore often concomitant with another disease. Pathogenic strains produce toxins that contribute to their ability to cause infection.

The organism remains viable for months in inanimate objects. Phage typing shows that poultry isolates are distinctive from mammalian and human types, and thus not cross-infective. Pathogenic strains will coagulate rabbit plasma and grow readily on common laboratory media. Particular phage types become endemic on a farm or in a geographic region. The organisms are moderately resistant to disinfectants.

Staphylococci bacteria are ubiquitous. They are always present in bird-producing facilities, especially buildings and ranges that are used repeatedly year to year. The organism is associated with the skin, common in the environment, and more prevalent in intensive bird-production areas. The incidence of the disease in birds grown on range or semiconfinement is five times that of birds reared in confinement.

TRANSMISSION AND CLINICAL SIGNS:

Staphylococcosis is an environmental disease often referred to as soilborne. It moves slowly through the flock because it does not spread from bird to bird. Any injury or break of epithelial surfaces, skin, or mucous membranes can be an entry site for infection. There are various manifestations of the disease, namely septicemia, arthritis, synovitis, osteomyelitis, and bumblefoot.

The incidence of staphylococcosis is higher in birds reared outdoors.

Birds contract the disease by drinking from stagnant pools in the yard. Mortality in untreated flocks may reach 15 percent but in treated flocks usually is less than 5 percent .

The disease becomes chronic if treatment is delayed or withheld and sick birds may linger for days to weeks. Clinical signs are sickness and inappetence, swollen joints, lameness, eye infections, emaciation, ruffled feathers, and diarrhea. Outbreak mortality is highest in birds 8 to 10 weeks of age.

Occasionally birds will develop wetness under the jaw. This is a cutaneous form of the disease. In septicemic form, the disease is similar to fowl cholera with depression, fever, and loss of appetite. Birds show pain on movement. The arthritic form usually follows the septicemic phase and lame birds develop swollen joints and breast blisters. Birds with bumblefoot have swollen abscessed footpads, a result of puncture wounds of the foot. Black rot may show up in eggs of infected hens because the organism can be passed into the egg.

LESIONS AND DIAGNOSIS:

With the septicemic form, the liver is swollen, congested, and greenish. Abdominal vessels are engorged with petechial hemorrhages on the heart, fat, and serosal surfaces. The skin becomes necrotic with thick exudates from birds with submaxillary lesions. In the arthritic forms, the joints become swollen and filled with creamy pus. Synovial membranes are thickened and edematous and foot lesions have thickened abscessed foot pads with caseous material.

In day-old hatchlings, a conjunctival form is observed in which the eye swells and mats shut. This infection comes through the hatching process. Gross diagnosis can be based on flock history, signs, and lesions. Confirmation is by isolation and identification of the pathogen. During necropsy, a gram stain of the exudate will show the presence of staphylococcal bacteria. The bacteria can be cultured from lesions of liver, eye, joint exudate, food pad, skin lesions, and bone marrow when osteomyelitis is present.

Additional laboratory tests such as the coagulase test are available when warranted. Treatment should be initiated on the basis of presumptive diagnosis, then altered if laboratory results show differently. An antibiotic sensitivity test should be requested on each laboratory submission.

TREATMENT AND CONTROL:

Staphylococcus aureus is sensitive to several antibiotics and some isolates are sensitive to sulfa drugs. Erythromycin, novobiocin, penicillin and tetracyclines are the most frequently prescribed medications. Other antibiotics such as lincomycin, spectinomycin, or LS-50 are beneficial when other antibiotics are not available. Tetracyclines and sulfa drugs are not consistently effective and should be used only when the isolate is test-sensitive to either of these drugs. Medication can be administered by feed or water (flock improvement is usually more rapid if medication is via drinking water) and should be continued for 5 to 7 days.

Vaccines against *S. aureus* are ineffective. An upgrading of sanitation, removal of hazardous conditions so as to protect birds from injury, and proper medication is good treatment regimen. Control depends on proper husbandry, housing, and nutrition with a reduction of stressors to provide a safe comfortable environment. Selenium and vitamin E levels in feed should be checked as these components are necessary for the tissues to maintain normal integrity. When selenium and vitamin are deficient, a condition called "exudative diathesis" (fluids under the skin) develops. Exudative diathesis makes the bird susceptible to *S. aureus* infections.

PREVENTION:

S. aureus is ubiquitous; therefore, its presence cannot be avoided. Prevention is achieved by providing special attention to flock care and general good husbandry, nutrition, along with equipment and pen maintenance. Remove objects that can cause injury to birds. Isolate chronically affected birds. Avoid the introduction of the infection when applying anti-pick devices. Prevent or reduce in-house dust. Be careful that the amount of selenium and other trace-elements in the feed is adequate.

STREPTOCOCCOSIS

DEFINITION:

Streptococcosis, a disease caused by a bacterium, is an acute to chronic infectious noncontagious disease of gamebirds, poultry, waterfowl, and wild birds. It occurs world-wide. The disease is characterized by septicemia, cyanosis, diarrhea, and high mortality. Other common names are strep and strep septicemia. The causative agent is *Streptococci*, a gram positive cocci that occurs singly, in pairs, and in chains, and are nonspore-forming, nonmotile, facultative anaerobes. Incubation requires 1 to 3 days and the course of the disease is 1 to 3 weeks. The most common species infecting birds are *S. zooepidemicus* and *S. faecalis* (referred to as fecal strip). Both are natural inhabitants of intestinal tracts of birds. Birds of all ages are susceptible but *S. zooepidemicus* is associated with infections of adult birds and *S. faecalis* infects embryos and young birds. *S. faecalis* in embryos and in hatchlings from fecally contaminated eggs is serious. The streptococcus of *S. faecium* and *S. mutans* are associated with mortalities in ducklings and goslings, respectively.

Streptococcosis is more serious where gamebirds are grown in confinement and the quality of sanitation lags. Birds of all types, mammals, and humans are susceptible but, like staphylococcus, the avian streptococci seldom cross-infects mammals and humans. Due to the low virulence of the organism, streptococci are considered as opportune pathogens that require simultaneous mitigating circumstances to produce the illness. Streptococci become host-adapted, which is why avian strains do not infect other animals or people. The organism will grow on laboratory media but growth is enhanced in a low-oxygen environment (facultative anaerobe).

TRANSMISSION AND CLINICAL SIGNS:

Streptococcus is normal intestinal microflora. Its transmission is linked to fecal contamination from feces or environment to host. Streptococcus, being an opportune pathogen, is associated with other contributing factors. The exception to this is egg contamination and septicemia in baby birds. Unsanitary environment provides the opportunity for infection to occur. Transmission is by the oral or respiratory aerosol routes. The severity of disease depends on the serotype of the pathogen and other prevailing circumstances. Septicemic birds are feverish and lethargic, and have pale combs. Egg production decreases or ceases and death occurs.

Chronically affected birds are sleepy, weak and lame, and have ruffled feathers. Diarrhea and head tremors appear; birds lose appetite and weight. Death occurs. Often the first clue of streptococcosis in the flock is the dead birds. Acute deaths may reveal few or no lesions, but birds that linger for a few days develop typical lesions. Egg transmission or fecal contamination of hatching eggs result in late embryo deaths, with increased numbers of chicks unable to "pip" or penetrate the shell to hatch. *S. faecalis* infected chicks develop endocarditis, detectable by listening (ear to ribs) for "snapping" or "clicking" sound produced by diseased heart valves. Affected chicks are visibly ill and death losses peak between 7 and 12 days of age.

LESIONS AND DIAGNOSIS:

Lesions in the acute disease form are nonspecific but include swollen liver and spleen with or without red, tan, or white foci; enlarged kidneys; and congestion of subcutaneous tissues, often with sanguinous and pericardial fluids and peritonitis. Omphalitis is observed in newly hatched birds. Chronic lesions include swollen joints with fibrinous synovitis, perihepatitis, pericarditis, necrotic myocarditis, and valvular endocarditis (clicking sound). The heart valve lesions are yellow, white, or tan with raised rough areas on the surface of the valve. The diseased heart is enlarged, pale, and flaccid. Other microscopic lesions are infarcts on myocardium, liver, spleen, lungs, kidney, and brain. The heart valve lesions show fibrin, bacteria and pus cells (heterophil WBC).

Chronic streptococcus infections focus particularly on the heart and kidneys. In humans, the condition is called rheumatic fever. History, clinical signs, and lesions suggest streptococcosis. Demonstration of bacteria in blood and heart valve-impression smears, and focal necrosis of other organs provide a presumptive diagnosis.

Disease confirmation irequires isolation and identification of the pathogen. Bacteria can be isolated from the heart blood, liver, and spleen lesions, tissue fluids, exudates, and yolk sac of chicks. The use of special culture media is helpful for species differentiation. Isolation and identification of known pathogenic strains confirms the diagnosis. Lesions may resemble those of other bacterial diseases, e.g., staphylococcosis, paratyphoid, colibacillosis, and fowl cholera. Serotype identification can be done by group-specific precipitin testing. Further tests are directed toward strain identification of the isolate.

TREATMENT AND CONTROL:

For optimal results, specific medication should be based on antibiotic-sensitivity tests made on the isolate obtained from the field case. Since streptococcus is a gram positive cocci, it is sensitive to penicillin, erythromycin, novobiocin, lincomycin, and gentamicin. Early in the course of the disease, clinically affected birds respond well to medication. Treatment efficacy decreases with progress and chronicity of the infection.

Novobiocin is recommended for ducks; with other birds, bacitracin in the feed as a preventive is helpful. Often times, medication selected for initial treatment will need to be changed during the course of treatment in order to control the outbreak. Streptococcus bacteria are capable of developing resistance to the drug in use. The caretaker must implement hygiene and sanitation measures and monitor flock mortality, progress of lesions, and other changes to provide effective control. The disease can relapse if medication is discontinued too soon or if unsanitary conditions prevail. Specific medication will minimize the course of the disease.

PREVENTION:

Correcting management practices, reducing stress, and preventing immunodepressive diseases are essential for preventing streptococcal infections. In severe outbreaks, growers should depopulate affected flocks, and totally decontaminate buildings, equipment, and pens. The use of recovered birds is risky, but feasible in order to preserve special genetic lines. Monitor the flock by regular laboratory culturing of embryos and cull birds for S. faecalis or other problematic streptococcal species. True prevention depends on biosecurity, flock hygiene, good nutrition, good husbandry, and good management.

ULCERATIVE ENTERITIS

DEFINITION:

Ulcerative enteritis, referred to as quail disease, is an acute bacterial infection of upland gamebirds, especially quail, chickens, and turkeys. The disease is caused by an anaerobic bacterium and is characterized by necrotic ulcerations in the intestine and cecum, and diffuse hepatic (liver) necrosis. The primary synonyms are UE and quail disease. The causative organism is *Clostridium colinum*, a soil-borne anaerobic, gram positive, spore-forming, rod-shaped bacterium. The organism is heat resistant and will withstand boiling for 3 minutes. Boiling is useful in destroying other contaminants during isolation procedures. *C. colinum* is fastidious in its growth requirement, needing enriched media and anaerobic conditions. The organism also grows in the yolk sacs of 5- to 7-day old chicken embryos. Because of its spore-forming ability, the anaerobe is resistant to germicides in the environment. The incubation period is 3 days in the acute form and 1 to 2 weeks in the chronic forms. The course of the disease is 2 to 6 weeks. UE occurs throughout the world and is diagnosed across the USA. Numerous reports have been recorded in Great Britain and Germany. Quail of all ages, especially those grown in captivity, are so susceptible to UE that producers must rear the birds on wire to control the disease. On-wire rearing prevents the exposure of birds to their feces, a principal source of the bacterium. Other gallinaceous birds are also susceptible, but less so than quail. On farms with UE problems, the organism will develop resistance to medication. Young birds are more susceptible than mature birds. Recovered birds remain carriers and shedders. Relapses of the disease often occur when birds are moved or undergo some other change in environment.

TRANSMISSION AND CLINICAL SIGNS:

UE is transmitted through droppings and birds become infected by ingesting contaminated feed, water, or litter. The organism produces spores that perpetually contaminate the premises after an outbreak. Interspecies transmission occurs among susceptible birds. Infection can spread mechanically on shoes, feed bags, equipment, and by flies, rodents, pets, and carrier birds. Infective spores live indefinitely in the environment; however, researchers consider the chronic carrier bird the primary factor of perpetuation. The disease is highly contagious among quail. The incubation period is 3 to 6 days and the course of the disease usually lasts 3 weeks, with the peak of mortality between the fifth and fourteenth days. Clinical signs include extreme depression; birds sit humped with eyes closed, have loss of appetite, ruffled feathers, and watery droppings; and become emaciated and die. In quail, the white watery feces is distinctive. In most species, early clinical signs are similar to those of coccidiosis. Early in the outbreak, sudden death may occur without any obvious signs as the birds may still be well fleshed. With quail, mortality in untreated flocks may range from 50 to 100 percent within a few days if the flock is not treated. More often the accumulated mortality ranges from 30 to 50 percent. In other species, mortality is much lower, ranging from 2 to 10 percent. As the disease becomes chronic, the flock is unthrifty and mortality continues for several days after treatment is initiated. The disease will relapse if medication is discontinued too soon, especially if the birds remain in a contaminated environment.

LESIONS AND DIAGNOSIS:

Lesions are similar in most birds. The primary lesions are found in the lower third of the small intestine, ceca, and liver. The intestinal lesions are yellow-white circular necrotic ulcerations. Deep ulcers can be seen through the unopened intestinal wall. Typical lesions have eroded centers that may perforate the intestinal wall. Other lesions are intestinal and cecal core formations, peritonitis, and intestinal adhesions. In chronically affected birds, the bacteria can be isolated from the liver. Liver lesions contain yellow to tan areas, focal yellow lesions or both. The spleen is swollen and hemorrhagic or necrotic and the muscle tissues are pale. A presumptive diagnosis can be based on history, clinical signs, and lesions. Stained intestinal impression smears reveal gram positive sporulated rod-shaped bacilli. Confirmation requires the isolation and identification of the agent *Clostridium colinum*. *C. colinum* is not always isolated but other clostridial bacteria may be recovered; therefore, the presence of any pathogenic clostridia is acceptable for a diagnosis of UE. Medication and hygiene are the same for all intestinal clostridial infections in gamebirds. Differential diagnosis is important to rule out coccidiosis, histomoniasis, trichomoniasis, and paratyphoid. Coccidiosis is often a complicating finding, in which case a judgment must be made whether it is the primary or secondary disease. With quail, UE (when present) should be the disease of primary concern even though both diseases will need immediate attention.

TREATMENT AND CONTROL:

The causative organism is susceptible to many antibiotics, especially those that work against gram positive bacteria. Bacitracin, neomycin, streptomycin, lincomycin, virginiamycin, and tetracycline are all effective against UE. Bacitracin and neomycin work together for initial medication; one is administered in the feed and the other in the drinking water. When mortality stops, discontinue the water treatment. Bacitracin dosage is 100 to 200 g/ton of feed and neomycin dosage is 200 mg/gal of water. Check for the legal levels for use of different drugs. Obey FDA withdrawal time for the drug before slaughter or release of treated birds. Control efforts (i.e., biosecurity, C& D) must continue beyond the medication period, as medicated birds have low resistance against reinfection. Replace contaminated litter and continue preventive medication. Consider rearing bob-white quail on wire. Add no new birds. Prevent contact with other species. Segregate young and old birds; do not mix birds of different ages. The pen remains infective until cleaned and disinfected, so upgrade pen sanitation and biosecurity.

PREVENTION:

UE is so difficult to prevent in quail that most growers ultimately maintain the birds on wire-bottom cages or pens. When quail have access to their droppings, UE eventually occurs. The usual hygienic precautions are vitally important. Likewise strict biosecurity is advised, not only for prevention of UE but for the prevention of other diseases. Management implies separate pens for birds by age and species, long known as good husbandry practice. Prevention of UE is best done by on-wire rearing; judicious use of medication; and uncompromising attention to good husbandry details, sanitation, and biosecurity.

GROWER'S REFERENCE

ON

GAMEBIRD HEALTH

III.   VIRAL DISEASES —105

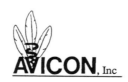

AVICON, Inc

AVIAN ENCEPHALOMYELITIS

DEFINITION:

Avian encephalomyelitis (AE) is an infectious viral disease characterized by incoordination and tremors of the head, neck, and limbs.
Avian encephalomyelitis, also called "epidemic tremors" or AE, was of
great economic importance until commercial vaccines became available in the 1960s. The causative agent is a picorna virus that can be
grown in chicken embryos from nonimmune hens. Incubation requires 10 to 17 days and the course of the disease is 2 to 4 weeks.
Physical, chemical, and serological tests demonstrate no significant
difference between the Van Roekel laboratory strain and the field isolates. Several avian species, especially chickens, coturnix quail, and
pheasant, are susceptible. Ducklings, pigeons, and guinea fowl are
susceptible to experimental infections.

AE occurs worldwide wherever poultry is raised. All flocks eventually
become infected with the virus. Clinical disease is low unless nonvaccinated breeders break with the disease during production. A survey
of breeder-replacement flocks revealed that 99 percent were positive
by 15 months of age. AE occurs in all seasons but most clinical cases
occur from January to June, the peak poultry-breeding period. The
pathogenicity of field isolates varies. All isolates are enterotropic;
young birds are readily infected when they ingest litter or feces contaminated by the isolate. The more "neurotropic" isolates cause
tremors in young birds. Most AE isolates cause paralysis in 18-day-old
embryos.

TRANSMISSION AND CLINICAL SIGNS:

The AE virus is transmitted through the egg from infected hens to the
chick during the viremic stage of infection in the hen. The disease
spreads laterally to hatch-mates in the hatcher and brooder. Infected
flocks experience low hatchability rates because embryos are paralyzed and unable to hatch. The hatch rate will be reduced for three
successive weekly hatches. Livability of chicks is decreased due to lateral spread. Lateral spread occurs from fecal contamination of the
feed and water by infected pen-mates. The onset of signs in hatchlings
occurs within 7 to 12 days. The virus can survive 4 weeks in droppings. Tremors of the head and neck are the primary clinical signs in
baby birds. Tremors can be exaggerated by shaking the bird. Affected
chicks show dull expression in the eyes, progressive incoordination,
tremors of head and neck, and finally paralysis. Other signs are inac-

tivity, reluctance to walk, or walking on hocks. All stages — dullness, tremors, and prostration — are seen in an outbreak. Birds lose weight because feed and water consumption decrease; however, many birds recover. Infected adult birds do not develop tremors or paralysis. Laying birds experience 5 to 20 percent drop in production with a corresponding drop in hatchability and chick livability. Morbidity reaches 60 percent and chick mortality 30 percent.

LESIONS AND DIAGNOSIS:

Gross lesions in young birds are obscure, but there may be whitish areas (clumps of WBC) in the muscle of the gizzard. Ocular hemorrhage and cataracts in semimature and mature birds are associated with AE. Microscopic lesions consist of lymphocytic foci in the pancreas, liver, gizzard, proventriculus, and brain. Brain lesions are described as perivascular cuffing with neuronal degeneration, endothelial hyperplasia, and gliosis. Brain lesions are further described as disseminated, nonpurulent encephalomyelitis and ganglionitis of the dorsal root ganglia. Leg muscles of AE-infected embryos are atrophied. The diagnosis of AE is based on a flock history of a drop in production and hatchability, higher mortality in hatchlings, chicks with tremors, weakness, and paralysis. There are no diagnostic gross lesions.

Confirmation is by one or more procedures such as fluorescent antibody test, virus isolation, chick transmission studies, agar gel precipitin test, and histopathology on pancreas, eye, liver, stomach, brain, and brain stem. The brain is an excellent tissue for isolation of the virus. Other infected tissues and organs will induce the disease when injected into chicks. AE must be differentiated from other encephalitic diseases, such as ND, EE, MD, encephalomalacia, and aspergillosis, or bacterial encephalitis.

TREATMENT AND CONTROL:

There is no specific treatment for acute outbreaks. Birds with clinical signs should be killed, and incinerated. Recovered chicks are unthrifty and the grower may be wise to opt to terminate the flock. If flock is not to be eliminated, a good nursing practice is to provide fresh feed and water throughout the outbreak, which runs 14 to 21 days in young flocks.

The period of virus passage from hen to eggs may last up to 6 weeks. Control is by vaccination of breeder-replacement birds during their growing period. Recovered breeders are immune, i.e., they no longer shed the virus. Inactivated vaccines are available and may be useful in flocks already in production. Live-virus vaccine after breeder flocks are in production would not be safe, because the virus would be transmitted to the chick.

PREVENTION:

AE is prevented only by the selection of eggs from immune breeder flocks. Lifetime immunity is achieved by recovery from a natural outbreak or by vaccination. For best immunity, vaccinate breeder replacement birds during their growing period, thus assuring that they do not become infected after maturity. Dissemination of the virus by the egg-borne route is thus prevented.

Maternal antibodies from the noncarrier hen protect progeny against contact with the AE virus during the critical first 3 weeks. A live embryo-propagated vaccine virus is recommended and is easily administered in the drinking water or by spray. Live-virus vaccines can be stored frozen or lyophilized. After administration, the virus will spread rapidly through the flock similar to the field virus. Withhold vaccination until the birds reach 6 weeks of age (or 4 weeks before onset of production).

AVIAN INFLUENZA

DEFINITION:

Avian influenza (AI) is a viral disease affecting the respiratory, enteric, or nervous systems of many bird species. The disease is characterized by respiratory signs, depression, and reduced feed and water consumption. Laying birds have a severe drop in egg production with reduced egg hatchability. The disease is called AI, flu, and influenza. AI is caused by any type A influenza virus, classified as an orthomyxovirus. The incubation period is 3 to 5 days and the course of the disease is 10 to 28 days. The virus type is determined by the cell wall antigens [Hemagglutinin (H) and Neuraminidase (N)]. There are 13 H and 9 N types identified in nature; all readily grow in avian species. The virus is sensitive to germicides and desiccation. AI virus remains viable for 103 days in liquid-manure systems and lake water inhabited by infected waterfowl. In warm weather, the virus remains viable for 21 days in poultry houses and longer in cool seasons. The virus hemagglutinates chicken RBC.

The most virulent form, once called fowl plague, is now called "Highly Virulent Influenza." Since the 1983-84 AI epidemic, terms describing AI as nonpathogenic, low-pathogenic, or highly pathogenic, (based on pathotyping of the isolate from an outbreak) have been used.

Pheasant, chukar, and Guinea fowl are the most susceptible of gamebird species. Waterfowl often are unaffected carrier-shedders. The viruses have worldwide distribution and are frequently recovered from clinically normal seabirds, migrating waterfowl, imported pet birds, and live-bird markets. AI is a reportable disease. State and federal regulatory agencies must be formally notified of any confirmed AI diagnosis.

TRANSMISSION AND CLINICAL SIGNS:

AI is readily spread by air currents, feces, humans, fomites, vehicles, flies, beetles, dead birds, and infected litter. Infected birds excrete virus in the feces. Experimentally, AI is transmissible by most routes of inoculation. Tropical birds are often a reservoir for AI that can spread to other caged birds, wild birds, and gamebirds. There is evidence that turkeys become infected with serotype H_1N_1 from pigs. The highly virulent H_5N_2 strain, cause of the 1983 Pennsylvania epidemic, must be reported to regulatory officials. Two clinical forms of AI have been described. The MILD form produces listlessness, respiratory involvement, diarrhea, and low mortality. The ACUTE form produces facial swelling, cyanosis, dehydration, and respiratory stress. The legs and comb may be dark red with whitish or ischemic areas. This is explained as blood pooling and tissue anemia within the same organ. The highly virulent form is ACUTE with a sudden onset, short course, morbidity and mortality near 100 percent. Sick birds act dazed, go off feed and water, and become cyanotic. Blisters form on combs and production drops to near zero with some shell-less eggs.

LESIONS AND DIAGNOSIS:

ACUTE AI produces severe septicemia. Lesions include hemorrhage, transudation, and necrosis in the respiratory and gastrointestinal tracts, skin, and urogenital system. Respiratory involvement is present to some degree in all AI outbreaks. Severely affected birds have greenish diarrhea, cyanosis, and swelling of the head, combs, and wattles. Hemorrhages appear on shanks and feet. The pharynx is blood stained and affected birds have a nasal discharge.

Sinusitis is common in quail, ducks, and turkeys. In acute outbreaks, mortality increases exponentially (perhaps 10 to 50 times that of the previous day). Mortality peaks (often reaching 70 to 100%) on the sixth or seventh day of illness.

Presumptive diagnosis can be based on flock history, clinical signs, and characteristic lesions. Confirmation requires isolation and identification of the virus and positive serology. Isolation of the virus in chicken embryos produces virus-laden allantoic fluid that will hemagglutinate chicken erythrocytes. Tissues for virus isolation include trachea, lung, exudates, liver, spleen, heart blood, and tracheal and cloacal swabs.

AI must be differentiated from Newcastle Disease, other paramyxoviruses, chlamydiosis, mycoplasmosis, and fowl cholera. The diagnostic laboratory or veterinarian on the case must report confirmed AI diagnosis to State and Federal disease regulatory officials.

TREATMENT AND CONTROL:

There is no practical specific medication for AI. Good husbandry with emphasis on hygiene and biosecurity to prevent spread is recommended. Recovery is rather spontaneous in birds mildly affected, but the disease is more devastating in acute cases. Birds slaughtered 7 days after recovery are free of lesions and show no significant increase in condemnation rate.

Several antiviral substances have been tried experimentally but have not been cleared, therefore they cannot be recommended. Killed vaccines are commercially available, but these are for use with exposed poultry rather than in treating outbreak flocks.

Many states allow the vaccines to be used only by permit. As part of the control program, infected premises should be placed under quarantine, either self-initiated by the grower or mandated by state authorities. Depopulated buildings and premises should be thoroughly cleaned and disinfected (C& D). Most states will provide a list of approved germicides, arrange for C& D with the producer, and supervise the C& D process. Poultry litter and manure must be composted before applying to cultivated land. This information is provided for the producer after AI has been confirmed in the flock.

PREVENTION:

Prevention is best accomplished by maintaining a closed flock and by practicing effective biosecurity. Nonresident birds, especially migratory waterfowl and seagulls, are the most likely source of the AI virus, but swine are susceptible to the H_1N_1 strain of AI and can also infect gamebirds.

Inactivated vaccines (autogenous) are helpful to prevent reoccurrence in exposed and replacement birds. Again, vaccines can be used only on approval. Vaccines are costly and their use is labor intensive. Each bird must be injected and then reinjected in 30 days. If a vaccination program is not undertaken, AI eradication under the auspices and supervision of state and/or federal regulatory officials is required.

AVIAN POX

DEFINITION:

Avian Pox is a slow-spreading viral disease of avian species, especially game, domestic, and wild birds. Pox in the DRY FORM is characterized by nodular skin lesions; in the WET FORM by diphtheritic throat lesions. Synonyms are AP, fowl pox, FP, quail pox, QP, sorehead, pigeon, canary, or parrot pox, and avian diphtheria.

Avian pox is caused by a large-DNA pox virus, an epitheliotropic virus. Incubation requires 4 to 10 days and the course of the disease is slow and extends for several weeks. There are eight (fowl, turkey, pigeon, canary, parrot, mynah, quail, and crane) or more known closely related, but distinguishable, pox viruses or strains. Perhaps all strains are host-modified, i.e., variants of what was once a single virus.

All pox viruses show identical morphology. The main components of the virus are protein, DNA, and lipid. The virus reproduces in the epithelial tissue (skin and mucus membranes). There is some cross immunity between strains. AP is not infectious to people. "Chicken pox" is a disease of humans, distinct from Avian Pox. AP virus is resistant in dry scabs. In laboratory cultures, the virus grows in certain tissue-culture cell lines and in the chorioallantoic membrane of chicken embryos.

Avian pox occurs worldwide. New pox species are being identified since larger numbers of wild, pet, and migratory birds are examined. Some isolates are host-specific, whereas other isolates will cross-infect different birds. The genomic profiles show differences from the typical fowl pox virus; therefore, pox infections are separate diseases requiring homologous vaccines for immune protection.

TRANSMISSION AND CLINICAL SIGNS:

AP is most likely introduced and transmitted into flocks by infected mosquitoes and blood-sucking arthropods; however, pox virus can transfer mechanically if in contact with injured or lacerated skin. Insects may deposit the virus in the eye. Eye lesions develop and/or the virus enters the mouth in tears swallowed that cause WET-FORM. DRY-POX is transmitted by infected mosquitoes. Transmission within flocks is rapid when mosquitoes are plentiful.

Eleven species of flying insects have been reported to be vectors of AP. The first recognized sign of pox is the presence of lesions on unfeathered parts of a few birds. Pox does not spread from bird to bird, so the course is usually slow and of long duration unless pox virus is within a building where transmission occurs by air. On range, AP is less acute because it is dependent on the mosquito as vector for spread. Only birds bitten by infected mosquitoes develop the pox lesion. The mortality is low. The wet or diphtheritic form develops when lesions occur in the upper respiratory or digestive tract. Lesions in the nasal cavity or eye (conjunctiva) produce nasal or ocular discharge similar to other infections or when birds eat AP-infected mosquitoes.

LESIONS AND DIAGNOSIS:

Typical pox lesions are diagnostic. The lesion is initially a raised, blanched, nodule that enlarges, turns yellowish, and progresses to form a thick dark scab. The lesion has been described as a proliferative wart-like cone-shaped nodule with a hollow center in which the scab is attached to the nodule with fibrin strands.

Cutaneous lesions occur on the unfeathered skin of face, head, vent, feet and legs. DIPHTHERITIC (WET-FORM) lesions are in the form of a false membrane in the mouth, esophagus, and trachea. In insect-induced outbreaks, WET-FORM lesions accompany the DRY FORM of the disease. The diphtheritic form can extend into the sinuses, upper throat, and nasal passages and obstruct breathing. In either form, the scab is firmly attached. A presumptive diagnosis can be based on typical skin and/or diphtheritic lesions. Confirmation is by isolation and identification of the pox virus supported by histopathological examination of the pox lesion.

Pox can be reproduced from lesion material inoculated into susceptible birds of the same species. The virus will grow and will produce lesions on dropped CA membranes of chicken embryos.

Lesions contain typical viral inclusion bodies. Histological confirmation is made by demonstrating intracytoplasmic viral inclusion bodies in stained sections or in scrapings from the lesions. Laryngeal and tracheal lesions must be differentiated from laryngotracheitis. Another confirmatory diagnostic procedure is electron microscopy. In most outbreaks, a diagnosis is made on gross and microscopic lesions and isolation of the virus.

TREATMENT AND CONTROL:

Flock vaccination with a homologous pox vaccine will stop the outbreak. In gamebirds, most pox outbreaks have been caused by quail pox (QP); therefore, QP-virus vaccine is recommended. Delay vaccinations until the birds are 8 weeks of age.

Vaccination of turkeys or chickens requires fowl pox, turkey pox, or pigeon pox vaccine. These three viruses offer some cross-protection against each other but not against quail pox. Most birds can be vaccinated by the wing web (WW) method, but birds that sleep with the head under the wing (as do turkeys) should be vaccinated on the leg by the feather-follicle method. Each bird must be vaccinated as the virus does not spread from bird to bird.

Recovery from the disease or vaccination confers lifetime immunity. AP is epitheliotropic; thus the vaccine must be inoculated into the skin (epithelium). The WW offers an ideal location for pox vaccination of most bird species.

Other control measures include mosquito control indoors by spraying dark areas (hiding places) with a poultry-use approved pesticide. Mow outside around the pens and apply an insecticide fog to kill or repel mosquitoes.

When pox vaccination fails to stop an outbreak, the most probable reason is that the wrong vaccine was used. QP has been reported in chickens in which FP offered no protection. Turkey pox vaccine should be used in wild turkeys or in flocks that are not protected by FP vaccines.

PREVENTION:

Pox vaccination is the only assured measure of protection. If pox is endemic, the birds should be vaccinated with a homologous vaccine to assure life-long protection. Mosquito-control programs reduce the bird's exposure to possible infected mosquitoes. Diphtheritic pox occurs first in the Spring because virus overwinters in mosquitoes and birds then feed on the emerging vectors.

DERZSY'S DISEASE

DEFINITION:

Derzsy's disease is a highly fatal acute parvovirus infection of wild and domestic goslings. The disease is characterized by septicemia, hepatitis, hydropericardium, ascites, feather loss, and anorexia. Derzsy's is also called goose parvovirus infection, goose influenza, goose plague, goose hepatitis, and ascitic hepatonephritis.

The causative agent is a parvovirus with no antigenic relationship to other animal parvoviruses. Its incubation period is 4 to 7 days and its course is 3 to 5 weeks. The virions are hexagonal. Virus replication occurs in the cell nucleus. Virus has been found in the heart and bursa of infected goslings. The virus is resistant to most germicides and is stable at pH 3 for 1 hour at 37°C. All goose parvovirus isolates are antigenically related.

The virus can be propagated in goose or muscovy embryos or primary cell cultures prepared from the embryos. All breeds of domestic and wild geese are susceptible, especially goslings and muscovy ducks. The disease is strictly age-dependent, with 100 percent mortality in birds younger than 1 week but with negligible losses in birds older than 4 weeks. Death occurs at 2 to 14 days (posthatch exposure) Mature birds seroconvert but show no clinical signs. Derzsy's disease has been reported in most countries of the world.

TRANSMISSION AND CLINICAL SIGNS:

The most serious outbreaks occur in susceptible goslings following vertical transmission of the virus. Infected birds excrete large amounts of virus in the feces. Transmission then occurs by direct and indirect contact. Recovered birds remain carriers and transmit the virus through their eggs to goslings in the hatchery.

Biological vectors have not been identified. Infected goslings are thirsty, inappetent, weak, reluctant to move, will huddle, and have profuse diarrhea. The disease progresses rapidly in goslings under one week of age that show anorexia and prostration. In the very young infected with the egg-passed virus, death occurs within 2 to 5 days. Mortality often reaches 100 percent.

Birds develop conjunctivitis and nasal discharge and tend to shake their heads. The uropygial glands and eyelids may be swollen. There may be abdominal ascites, forcing birds to assume a penguin-like posture. Goslings become stunted and lose down from areas around the neck and back. The disease is more protracted in older birds or in those with maternal antibodies. Complicating factors such as poor hygiene, secondary bacterial, fungal, or other viral infections will boost the final mortality.

LESIONS AND DIAGNOSIS:

During the peracute stage, an extensive fibrinous pseudomembrane is present over the tongue, mouth, and esophagus of the duckling or gosling.

Other common lesions are found in the heart, which becomes rounded with pale myocardium. The liver, spleen, and pancreas are swollen and congested. Typically, a serofibrinous perihepatitis and pericarditis are present. These birds are the ones with abdominal ascites. In longer-standing cases, there is pulmonary edema, liver atrophy, muco-catarrhal enteritis, and an enlarged thyroid. Histological lesions include focal degeneration of heart and liver, muscle necrosis, and hemorrhage with fatty accumulations in the liver. Other lesions are heterophilic infiltration, bile-duct proliferation, and intranuclear inclusions in the Kupffer's cells.

A presumptive diagnosis can be based on history of onset, course, age of birds, mortality, and lesions. Confirmation is by virus isolation in susceptible goose or muscovy duck embryos and tissue cultures. Other diagnostic tests are viral neutralization, fluorescent antibody, and electron microscopy. Differential diagnoses include duck virus enteritis, duck virus hepatitis, avian influenza, hemorrhagic nephritis, and enteritis. Infections of bacteria such as *Pasteurella (Riemerella) anatipestifer* and *E. coli* should also be considered. Many of the differential diseases are capable of producing lesions similar to those described.

TREATMENT AND CONTROL:

There is no treatment specific for Derzsy's Disease. Antibiotic therapy is helpful in control of losses from secondary infections. Strict isolation of susceptible goslings and ducklings is imperative during their first 4 weeks. Immunization of the breeders will elevate the level of maternal antibodies to provide some protection for 21 to 28 days, the critical period. The virus is attenuated by 40 passages in goose fibroblast tissue culture.

Do not mix eggs of different breeds in the incubator and hatcher. Set only eggs from known parvovirus-free breeders, because the disease is confined to young geese or muscovy ducklings. A biosecurity program is essential. Serum therapy or passive immunization is practiced in Europe, using serum from hyperimmunized geese. Two doses are required. This procedure is expensive and is recommended only for outbreak situations. Control requires good husbandry, isolation, and segregation of birds by age. NEVER ADD NEW HATCHES TO AN INFECTED FACILITY.

Pick up and incinerate dead goslings. Obtain a laboratory diagnosis early during an outbreak. Do not save recovered birds as breeders. On infected premises, immunize future breeder replacement birds with the live attenuated vaccine. Use only inactivated vaccines on parvovirus-free farms.

PREVENTION:

Disease eradication and vaccination are the surest ways to control and to prevent goose parvovirus infection. Eradication requires the total depopulation of the premises, thorough C& D of buildings, pens, and equipment. Leave pens empty for 30 to 90 days, or until the next production year.

Replace birds from known parvovirus-free sources. Tighten biosecurity to further prevent reintroduction. The other choice is to initiate a vaccination program, using attenuated vaccines initially, and inactivated vaccines later. Simultaneously upgrade basic care, sanitation, and management for birds of all ages. Recovered birds do remain carriers but the hens pass on passive immunity. In any event, eradication should be the ultimate goal.

DUCK VIRUS ENTERITIS

DEFINITION:

Duck virus enteritis is an acute, highly contagious herpes virus infection of ducks, geese, and swans. The disease is characterized by vascular damage, tissue hemorrhages, free blood in the abdominal cavity, and proliferative diphtheritic lesions of the digestive tract mucosa. Synonyms are DVE and duck plague. Incubation requires 3 to 7 days and the disease runs its course in 3 to 4 days. Sick ducks show sudden onset of weakness and incoordination, followed quickly by death.

The virus grows in the chorioallantoic (CA) membrane of susceptible duck or chicken embryos. DVE strains, though identical immunologically, vary in pathogenicity. The virus produces intranuclear inclusion bodies in a variety of cells in infected birds. Waterfowl of all ages are susceptible; in young birds, morbidity will be nearly 100 percent and mortality will range from 5 to 60 percent. Muscovy ducks appear to be the most susceptible, and mortality in adult ducks often reaches 100 percent.

DVE was first reported in the Netherlands, in 1923. Now it has been reported in most of the major duck-producing areas of the world. In 1967, DVE first appeared in white Peking ducks raised commercially on Long Island, NY. DVE has not been reported in nonanseriforme bird species. DVE has caused high mortality in wild waterfowl in major USA migratory flyways.

TRANSMISSION AND CLINICAL SIGNS:

DVE is transmitted parenterally, intranasally, or orally. The virus is also transmitted by contact with infected birds or environment. The virus is spread by infected droppings in feed, water, pools, ponds, and waterways. DVE virus enters the mucosa of mouth, nose, cloaca, and skin wounds as the bird eats, drinks, or swims. Infected birds remain carriers for as long as one year. Population densities in concentrated duck-producing areas contribute to the rapid spread of DVE.

Blood-sucking arthropods may also spread the disease as they feed on viremic birds. In young domestic ducklings, DVE clinical signs appear within 3 to 7 days following exposure. When overt signs appear, death follows within 1 to 5 days. Natural infection has been observed in ducks of all ages, ranging from ducklings to mature breeders. In domestic breeders, sudden high persistent mortality is usually the first observation. Mature ducks die in good flesh. Sick birds show inappetence, weakness, ataxia, photophobia, matted eyelids, nasal discharge, thirst, and diarrhea. The bird becomes exhausted and unable to stand.

As weakness increases, the bird balances itself with outstretched wings with its head down. Most birds with clinical signs die, often seeking isolation in vegetation near water. Typical death position is sternal with the beak into the earth. Dead male birds have prolapse of the penis. As DVE progresses, many birds have soiled vents and ruffled feathers. Young ducklings, 2 to 7 weeks of age, show dehydration, weight loss, blue beaks, and blood-stained vents.

LESIONS AND DIAGNOSIS:

Hemorrhages are present at many sites and there may be free blood in body cavities, gizzard, or intestine. Destruction of lymphoid tissues and degenerative changes in the organs will be seen. Hemorrhages are present on the heart, liver, pancreas, and mesenteries. Hemorrhage and necrosis are extensive throughout the body.

A diphtheritic membrane develops along the gastrointestinal tract. Elevated crusty plaques are present in the esophagus, ceca, rectum, and cloaca or bursa of Fabricius. In young birds, the esophageal mucosa may slough. There is hemorrhage and necrosis in the intestinal annular bands in ducks or lymphoid discs of geese. The spleen is normal or shrunken. The liver is discolored, hemorrhagic, and bile stained with multiple white foci. All lymphoid tissues are affected.

Ruptured yolks and free blood may be found in the abdominal cavity of laying duck hens. A presumptive diagnosis of DVE is based on flock history, signs, typical lesions, and epizootic losses. The gross lesions are generally diagnostic for DVE. Histologically, there are intranuclear inclusions in liver hepatocytes and mucosa of the digestive tract. Other diagnostic tests are virus neutralization and fluorescent antibody procedures.

Virus isolation and identification can be used to confirm the diagnosis. Virus isolation is done by inoculation of duck embryo fibroblasts, or the CA membrane of 9- to 14-day-old duck embryos. DVE in domestic flocks is reportable to State Regulatory and Department of Natural Resource (DNR) officials. Upon consideration of the situation, officials may choose to do nothing. Or they may quarantine and depopulate the flock. When the total flock dies because of DVE, there is usually no followup action by poultry health officials.

TREATMENT AND CONTROL:

Medication is not successful. The disease is self-limiting in flocks if new birds are not added. Early diagnosis, strict sanitation, and good husbandry will minimize losses.

Control measures include flock quarantine, strict biosecurity, and preventing resident birds from commingling with wild waterfowl. A commercial vaccine is available, but in many states legal use is by permit only.

Long-term control first requires eradication of the disease, then maintenance of DVE-free birds in an environment free of the virus. This may be difficult in premises located near streams and lakes visited by wild waterfowl.

Once DVE is present, control requires depopulation, thorough C&D, and exclusion of all waterfowl from the premises for 30 days or longer. In states where DVE is reportable, the authorities decide how to control the outbreak. The regulatory officials supervise C&D procedures. The producer is advised to contact the appropriate officials before initiating costly procedures that may have to be repeated.

PREVENTION:

Prevention is by establishing and maintaining a DVE-free flock. An outbreak requires eradicating the disease from the premises and restocking with birds from DVE-free sources when it is safe to do so.

Repair buildings and make other needed environmental changes to keep your waterfowl away from waters frequented by wild ducks and geese.

Establish a strict biosecurity program. Investigate the use, where permitted, of a vaccine for replacement birds. Employ all good husbandry and management practices.

DUCK VIRUS HEPATITIS

DEFINITION:

Duck Virus Hepatitis is a contagious, rapidly spreading, and highly fatal disease of young ducklings. The disease is characterized by a short incubation period, sudden onset, rapid course, development of characteristic liver lesions, and high mortality. The usual synonym is DVH. The causative agent is a picorna virus, a small RNA virus. Three distinct serotypes have been isolated from infected ducklings.

Serotype I has an incubation period of 18 to 48 hours, and has caused a natural outbreak in Mallard ducks. The course of the disease is 3 to 4 days. The virus is rather stable and difficult to eliminate from infected premises. Serotype I virus becomes noninfectious after the 20th serial passage in chicken embryos.

Ducklings from immune breeders withstand the infection for 3 to 6 weeks. Recovered birds are immune. This virus can also be isolated from the liver of experimentally infected poultry. Experimentally, DVH Type I infection has been produced in goslings, turkey poults, young pheasants, quail, and guinea fowl.

DVH Type II virus is now classified an astrovirus.

DVH Type III is reclassified as a picornavirus. Both II and III are antigenically distinct from DVH Type I. Ducks are the only natural host of DVH Type I and the virus primarily affects ducklings younger than 3 weeks. Adult ducks are not affected; there is no drop in egg production or fertility. DVH was first reported on Long Island, NY. Now the disease is recognized in all duck-raising areas of the world. In the United States, DVH remains one of the major diseases of the duck production industry.

TRANSMISSION AND CLINICAL SIGNS:

DVH can be transmitted by parenteral and by oral administration. Field experience with Type I virus indicates that egg transmission does not occur. DVH is highly contagious within the pen but does not spread easily to nearby pens. The virus is excreted in the feces of recovered ducklings for 8 weeks after onset of the disease. Transmission occurs primarily by ingestion of contaminated feed or water, or when the environment is contaminated. Experimentally, the disease has been spread by aerosols, but natural spread is thought to be mostly by ingestion. The portal of the entry is the pharynx or upper respiratory tract. Virus administered by capsule failed to produce infection.

Wild birds are capable of spreading the disease over short distances, but recent findings suggest that rats and other rodents act as reservoirs on infected premises. Affected ducklings become lethargic, lie on their side with heads drawn back, and paddle their feet spasmodically. Death follows within 30 minutes. The onset of signs is sudden and the course within the flock is 3 to 4 days. Mortality in ducklings younger than 3 weeks may reach 95 percent. Progressive symptoms are weakness, squatting, partial closing of the eye, incoordination, convulsions, and death. The death position is with legs extended backwards and head over back (opisthotonos). Mortality is age related, being highest in younger ducklings. In older or parentally immune ducklings, incidence of clinical signs and losses may be so low that the disease may go unnoticed.

LESIONS AND DIAGNOSIS:

The cadaver may be in opisthotonos position and have a greatly swollen mottled liver, enlarged spleen and kidneys, with congestion of the renal artery and viscera. Older ducklings show pericarditis, air sac infection, and white to yellow discharges. Microscopic changes in the acute disease are characterized by extensive necrosis of the hepatocyte cytoplasm and wide-spread bile duct hyperplasia. A presumptive diagnosis is based on history, lesions, and disease pattern, course (sudden onset, rapid spread, and acute), high mortality in younger ducklings, typical lesions, virus isolation, and the absence of bacteria. The virus can usually be isolated in 9- to 11-day chicken or duck embryos and day-old ducklings. The liver is the preferred organ for virus isolation. Once the virus is isolated, it can be identified and serotyped by virus neutralization, using DVH-specific antiserum. The disease must be differentiated from duck virus enteritis, Newcastle Disease, and avian influenza. DVH virus does not agglutinate RBC, a diagnostic feature of ND and AI. The death position of the duckling is characteristic and diagnostic for DVH.

TREATMENT AND CONTROL:

DVH does not respond to antibiotic therapy. If available, the only beneficial treatment is the use of DVH-specific antiserum collected from recovered or immunized birds at the time of slaughter. Antiserum may be available from the Duck Disease Laboratory, Eastport, Long Island, NY 11931. Serum-induced protection lasts only 3 days. Treatment involves the intramuscular injection of each duckling with 0.5 ml of antiserum. Do not treat until signs of DVH appear. An alternative to the use of the antiserum is the use of yolk material from eggs produced by hyperimmune breeder ducks or by hyperimmunized specific-pathogen-free (SPF) chickens.

PREVENTION:

At onset of the problem, administer antiserum or egg-yolk antibodies to all susceptible ducklings. Unexposed ducklings can be vaccinated using a chicken-embryo-adapted attenuated vaccine. Ducklings younger than 3 weeks of age may not respond to vaccination if they have maternal antibodies.

Immunize breeders with DVH-attenuated vaccine. Many producers revaccinate breeding ducks at 3- to 4-week intervals so as to maintain high maternal antibody titers. The progeny retain immunity for 3 to 6 weeks, after which DVH causes minimal health problems.

Natural DVH outbreaks in Mallard ducks have been reported, even though the Peking ducks are the most susceptible. Flock isolation and effective biosecurity are important strategies in every disease prevention and health program of gamebirds.

EQUINE ENCEPHALITIS

DEFINITION:

Equine encephalitis is an acute contagious disease of pheasants that also affects chukars, turkeys, ducks, pigeons, and wild birds. The disease is characterized by neurological signs related to microscopic lesions in the brain and spinal cord. There is usually an absence of major gross lesions. Synonyms include EE, EEE, WEE, and equine encephalomyelitis.

The causative agent, togaviridae, can be any one of the viruses classified as arboviruses. These viruses are able to infect hematophagous (blood-feeding) arthropods and are so similar that they are classified as Group A arboviruses. Nonetheless, the equine encephalitis viruses are separate, distinct, and share only minor antigenic components, and therefore are easily distinguished by serological methods. Incubation requires 2 to 5 days and the course of the disease is 2 to 4 weeks.

Arboviruses also vary in virulence. The eastern equine encephalitis is the most pathogenic. The virus reproduces in the arthropod and is transmitted when this vector then bites the bird or animal host. Mosquitoes are the primary vector to spread EE. *Aedes, Culex,* and *Mansonia* species are primary vectors to mammals. *Culiseta malinura* is the vector associated with transmitting EE to birds since *C. malinura* feeds only on birds.

Birds were thought to be reservoir hosts, but recent work has shown that the arbovirus overwinters in the mosquito or arthropod vector and not in the definitive host. Birds of all ages are susceptible; but the disease is more often diagnosed in older birds that, by being out of doors, have a greater risk of exposure.

EE occurs throughout the United States. The virus has been isolated from mice, rats, foxes, dogs, and other mammals. EE is highly infectious to people.

TRANSMISSION AND CLINICAL SIGNS

EE is introduced and principally spread by infected vectors. Mosquitoes and other blood-feeding arthropods are the vectors for EE. Spread of the disease within the pen occurs when susceptible birds cannibalize sick and viremic birds. The disease can occur indoors, but usually only birds kept out of doors are affected. The clinical signs of the various EE forms are similar; however, the clinical signs of central nervous system disturbance varies with different species of birds. In pheasants, there is a pronounced leg paralysis, torticollis (head over back), and tremors. There is a high mortality of chukars. Turkeys become drowsy, weak, paralyzed, then die. In all birds, signs include ataxia, leg and neck paralysis, inability to stand, and presence of tremors.

Few birds with these signs will recover. Accumulated flock mortality can be up to 95 percent, but is usually less. EE-infected ducks have posterior paresis, paralysis, and death with mortality up to 60 percent. Most signs are neurological in origin, reflecting brain damage caused by the viral encephalitis.

LESIONS AND DIAGNOSIS:

There are no significant gross lesions. Microscopic lesions are confined to the central nervous system, brain, spinal cord, and spinal nerves. Brain tissue of the clinically affected bird is the tissue of choice to demonstrate microscopic lesions. The lesions are not diagnostic in and of themselves because they resemble those of other viral encephalitic diseases. A presumptive diagnosis can be based on the history of onset within the flock (season and presence of mosquitoes), absence of gross lesions, and the presence of typical microscopic lesions. Confirmation is made by positive serological tests, virus isolation, and identification.

Caretakers, diagnosticians, and laboratory workers must exercise precautions to avoid exposure or inhalation of aerosols when handling birds. EE is a serious public health disease. EE-suspect cases must be reported to animal disease regulatory officials. Most state laboratories will not do virus isolation on suspect tissues. Therefore, all diagnostic materials should be sent to the USDA National Veterinary Services Laboratory, Ames, IA. EE must be differentiated from other forms of encephalitis, namely ND, AE, aspergillosis, botulism, mycotoxicosis, and encephalomalacia.

TREATMENT AND CONTROL:

Treatment of sick birds is without value. Remove the source of infection by establishing mosquito control. Keep a 50-foot strip of the vegetation around the building and pens cleared, thus destroying mosquito resting areas. Eliminate as many mosquito breeding places as possible. Keep shorelines of ponds and lakes mowed to remove vegetation (again, mosquito resting areas). Fog areas with malathion or other pesticides effective against mosquitoes. All pesticides must be

FDA approved for use on poultry.

Promptly remove and kill clinically affected birds to prevent cannibalism. Incinerate or bury dead birds. Burial must be adequately deep (at least 4 feet) to discourage digging by dogs or wild carnivores. Wear protective clothing and leather gloves in handling sick and dead birds. Establish pen isolation as much as possible by practicing strict sanitation between and within pens.

PREVENTION:

The most practical approach to protect birds from mosquitoes is outlined above. Develop an effective program to control cannibalism. Control external parasites, lice, and mites; presence of these pests on the premises often leads to feather picking and cannibalism.

An equine encephalitis vaccine that can be used to protect valuable blood lines is commercially available. Do not vaccinate birds younger than 6 weeks. Use vaccines in accordance with manufacturers' instructions. Keep records of flocks vaccinated, date, brand of vaccine, lot, and serial number. Mosquito control is the most important aspect of a prevention program. Public health officials can generally provide information and advice on mosquito control and the EE situation in your area.

INCLUSION BODY HEPATITIS

DEFINITION:

Inclusion-body hepatitis (IBH) is an acute infectious disease of quail, turkeys, and chickens. IBH is caused by an adenovirus and is characterized by sudden onset, sharply increased mortality, pathologic liver changes, anemia, and intramuscular hemorrhage. The incubation period is 1 to 3 days and the course of the disease is 10 to 13 days. The name of the disease is descriptive of the lesions. The disease is also called IBH, aplastic anemia, and hemorrhagic syndrome.

At least three serotypes of adenovirus have been isolated. Other adenovirus infections include quail bronchitis and marble spleen disease. The virus can be isolated from liver, spleen, kidney, and bursa of Fabricius. IBH is often associated with other predisposing conditions, e.g., infectious bursal disease. Adenoviruses are resistant and persist in contaminated facilities. Young gamebirds are the primary host, but Type I adenoviruses can be recovered from pigeons, mallard ducks, budgerigars, turkeys, and Guinea fowl.

IBH is clinically undetectable in breeder or adult flocks. Adenovirus infections in adult birds usually show up as mild transient respiratory infections. IBH infections are reflected in lower hatchability of fertile eggs and increased mortality in hatchlings. Adenoviruses are ubiquitous and reported worldwide, especially in major poultry producing areas. A variety of maladies of avian species are caused by members of the family of adenoviruses.

TRANSMISSION AND CLINICAL SIGNS:

Adenoviruses are transmitted both vertically (i.e., in the egg) and horizontally (to contact penmates). Horizontal spread occurs from direct contact with infected birds and with contaminated feed, water, and litter. High mortality and condemnation in broilers occurs when the viral infection is complicated with secondary bacterial super infections, especially those by *E. coli* and clostridial organisms.

High-virus fecal shedding is associated with stress periods in the life of the bird. Virus is also present in the trachea, nasal secretions, and renal urates, but the feces is the primary route of elimination.

Prevalent signs are sudden onset, depression, fever, and mortality that increases for 3 to 5 days. Then dying levels off for 3 to 5 days, and then decreases to preoutbreak rates after another 3 to 5 days. Losses from the disease approach 10 percent. The course of the disease averages 10 to 13 days. Day-old chicks from infected breeders are anemic. Packed cell volumes in individual chicks may be 12 percent (normal value: approximately 35%). There are few specific signs. Subtle signs include pale combs, wattles, and facial skin. The birds are depressed and listless.

LESIONS AND DIAGNOSIS:

The primary lesions are circulatory in nature and include anemia and jaundice with pale skin and bone marrow. Other gross lesions include swollen, congested, mottled liver, fibrinous perihepatitis, enlarged spleen and kidneys, and hemorrhage in muscles and organs. Microscopically, there is extensive degeneration and necrosis in the liver with intranuclear inclusions in hepatic cells and hypoplasia of bone marrow (aplastic anemia). The hepatocellular inclusions occur during the acute phase of the disease and persist for 3 days. Most of the affected birds are well fleshed.

A tentative diagnosis is based on history, symptoms, and gross lesions along with absence of other diseases. Demonstration of intranuclear inclusions is often used as the basis for a diagnosis. The adenovirus can be isolated from the respiratory and digestive tracts as well as from the liver. The agar gel precipitation test is used to demonstrate the presence of antibodies. Virus isolation is done in chicken embryos. IBH virus-induced embryo mortality occurs from 5 to 10 days after inoculation. Dead embryos are hemorrhagic and have focal necrosis with typical hepatic inclusions. Convalescent birds are seropositive. Differential diagnoses include campylobacter (vibrio) infection and mycotoxicosis.

TREATMENT AND CONTROL:

There is no effective medication. Good husbandry and care help to minimize mortality. Antibiotics will control bacterial infections and vitamins C and K help control the anemia and hemorrhage. In progeny from IBH-suspect breeders, medication should be given 2 to 3 days before anticipated IBH outbreak (based on previous outbreaks). Repeat medication in the next four to five hatches. Three days of supplemental iron, copper, and cobalt compounds will speed recovery from the anemia. Control is focused on elimination of the prevailing outbreaks and includes upgrading sanitation, bird comfort, and general biosecurity.

PREVENTION:

Thorough C& D of all brooding facilities. Biosecurity and good sanitary practices are the best defense against IBH. Keep wild birds out of the brooding and rearing buildings, as wild birds can transmit adenovirus to gamebirds and poultry. No vaccine is available.

Incidence of acute IBH has decreased. Vaccination for and control of immunosuppressive diseases will decrease the severity of IBH. In gamebirds, quail bronchitis and marble spleen diseases are the precursor diseases to IBH infection because of their immunodepressive action.

LARYNGOTRACHEITIS

DEFINITION:

Laryngotracheitis (LT) is a highly acute, contagious viral respiratory disease of several avian species. LT is caused by a virus that is characterized by respiratory distress and bloody tracheal exudates. Other names include LT, Trach, and Laryngo. The causative agent is a herpes virus that has an incubation period of 2 to 12 days. The course of the disease is 7 to 14 days. The virus remains alive and potent when frozen but is easily destroyed by germicides and direct sunlight. It survives for long periods in tissue exudates and materials such as expectorated tracheal clots and in carcasses of birds dead from the disease. All are carry-over sources on the farm.

There appears to be only one immunologic virus strain, though isolates vary in their pathogenicity. Most isolates tend to be pathogenic and cause the disease. The virus can be propagated in chicken embryos and certain tissue cell lines. LT virus infection produces Type A intranuclear inclusion bodies in respiratory epithelial tissues. Chickens are the most susceptible of the avian species, but LT is known to cause problems in pheasants and has been reported in peafowl. Juvenile and adult birds are the natural ages affected. The virus has been able to adapt and infect birds of broiler age. LT has been reported in most of the intensive poultry producing areas of the USA and many other countries.

TRANSMISSION AND CLINICAL SIGNS:

Natural infection routes are the upper respiratory tract and the ocular conjunctiva. Spread of LT is slower than that of other respiratory diseases. LT can be contracted by ingestion. Once it enters the flock, LT spreads by bird-to-bird contact or by bird contacting infected tissue, dead infected birds, infected environment, or through the administration of nonattenuated vaccines. Mechanical transmission occurs via contaminated clothing, shoes, tires, and other fomites. Recovered birds remain carriers for 24 months. New LT cases have been traced to poultry farm helpers. Because of faulty biosecurity, LT has spread from contaminated live-haul trucks and crates, especially those servicing the chicken industry.

Frequently, the first noticeable sign is birds with watery eyes. Affected birds remain quiet because breathing is difficult. There is marked dyspnea, often with loud gasping sounds. Other signs include coughing, sneezing, and shaking of the head (in trying to dislodge plugs in the trachea), and the expectoration of bloody mucus.

Affected birds extend the neck with mouth open to breathe, and wheeze when they inhale. Many birds die from asphyxiation due to blockage of the trachea. Mortality can be as high as 70 percent. The average mortality in chickens is 10 to 20 percent, but in pheasant and peafowl it is considerably lower.

The duration of the disease in the flock is up to 6 weeks. Individual birds die within 6 to 10 days; if not, they will usually recover. All birds in the flock become infected eventually. In caged birds, LT may appear as an outbreak with a relapse because on the first passage through the flock, not all birds contracted LT. On second passage, the remaining susceptible birds become infected.

LESIONS AND DIAGNOSIS:

Lesions occur most consistently in tracheal and laryngeal tissues. As named, the dominant lesion is severe laryngotracheitis with bloody exudates, initially in the trachea. As the disease progresses, blood-tinged exudates are evident and diphtheritic membranes form in the trachea and pharynx. The exudates of the pharynx wipe off easily in contrast to wet pox, in which exudates adhere and leave a raw bleeding surface. Characteristic false membranes in trachea and pharynx are diagnostic. A presumptive diagnosis can be based on flock history, clinical signs, and gross lesions.

Diagnosis is confirmed by virus isolation and identification. Absences of lesions in other organs and tissues are of diagnostic value. Diagnostic procedures include fluorescent antibody test, virus isolation, histopathologic examination, and demonstration of virus inclusions in respiratory epithelium and tracheal mucosa. The virus grows in the chorioallantoic (CA) membrane of chicken embryos. Histologically, the virus inclusions can be demonstrated to confirm the diagnosis.

TREATMENT AND CONTROL:

LT is a reportable disease. Treatment must include flock or farm quarantine and tight biosecurity. Implement control measures that include a separate caretaker for the sick flock, with no cross-traffic to other poultry. Upgraded sanitation and prompt incineration of dead birds are critical functions, as is careful administration of antibiotics.

Mass vaccination by spray or drinking water method is recommended for large commercial or caged flocks. In smaller flocks, vaccinate birds individually by the eye-drop method. Often the tracheal exudates plug can be removed with a swab.

Control relies upon management strategies to prevent spread and to enhance comfort of the bird. Do not add LT-recovered, -vaccinated, or -exposed birds to a susceptible flock.

Eradication of the disease requires depopulation, thorough C& D of the premises, and leaving buildings and pens empty for 4 to 6 weeks.

An alternate program involves annual flock vaccination with an attenuated LT vaccine.

PREVENTION:

To prevent LT, maintain good biosecurity. Always practice good husbandry concerning environment, feed, and sanitation. On infected premises, vaccinate replacement birds annually. LT vaccination is part of a total flock-vaccination program. Young birds should be vaccinated when 7 weeks of age. Birds vaccinated earlier should be revaccinated at 7 weeks.

Even though immunity is considered lifelong, exhibition (i.e., show) birds should be revaccinated annually because of the high exposure potential. Use attenuated nonspreading vaccines only. Do not mix vaccinated birds with nonvaccinated flocks. The quarantines imposed by state regulatory officials prevent the spread of LT to other farms.

MARBLE SPLEEN DISEASE

DEFINITION:

Marble Spleen Disease (MSD) is a contagious viral disease of ringneck pheasants that is characterized by the swollen and "marbling" appearance of the spleen, swollen liver, pulmonary congestion, and death. Synonyms are marble spleen, MSD, and lung edema. Marble spleen is caused by a Type II adenovirus serologically related to hemorrhagic enteritis (HE) of turkeys. At the peak of infection, the virus concentrates in the spleen.

Marble spleen disease virus can be propagated in turkey poults. In experimentally induced infections, maximal lesions occurred 6 to 7 days after inoculation. Serotypes of varying virulence probably exist in nature. Marble spleen is likely to occur in alternate years on infected farms. One explanation for this is that parental immunity from immune breeders shields the progeny from the disease.

Outbreaks of the disease seldom hit all pens on a farm. Incubation in experimental infections required from 6 to 8 days and the course of the disease was 1 to 3 weeks. Pheasants of all ages are susceptible. Mortality is greatest in birds 10 to 12 weeks or older. MSD occurs only in domestically grown pheasants and is not a serious threat to noncaptive birds.

Recovered birds appear to be immune for life. Morbidity is thought to be 100 percent in pens experiencing an outbreak. Mortality in these pens ranges from 5 to 15 percent, depending on environment and other factors. An outbreak often stops spontaneously after spreading to three or four pens.

Marble spleen is reported in the northeastern United States, Canada, and Italy. It is, however, probably much more widespread. Now that its cause is known and diagnostic procedures have been developed, reports from other pheasant-producing areas in the world are anticipated.

TRANSMISSION AND CLINICAL SIGNS:

The disease spreads from ingested infected material from feed or water and from bird to bird by pecking. Experimentally induced infections have been consistently produced by intravenous or oral inoculations of splenic extract. The spleen of an MSD-infected pheasant usually weighs four times that of normal pheasants (2.25 g vs 0.66 g). Based on research, the natural route of infection is by mouth. Clinical signs are vague.

Sudden unexplained death is the first clue and the only outward sign. Affected birds are thrifty and well-fleshed when found dead. Dead birds must be autopsied to determine actual cause of death. If marble spleen disease, typical lesions will be present. Death is caused by pulmonary stress. Affected birds suffocate from hemorrhage and edema of the lungs. The course of the disease ranges from 1 to 3 weeks within the outbreak pen; duration on the farm is normally from 6 to 8 weeks. The average cumulative mortality on affected farms is 8 to 12 percent, with mortality ranging from 5 to 15 percent within some pens.

LESIONS AND DIAGNOSIS:

Typical gross lesions include swelling and marbling of the spleen, hemorrhage and edema of the lungs, and swelling of the liver. Microscopic lesions include intranuclear inclusion bodies in lymphatic cells and the presence of necrotic areas in the lungs, spleen, and Kupffer's cells of the liver (focal necrotic areas abound in these three organs). Lymphocytic aggregates are found in the proventriculus.

Electron microscopic examination of splenic cells reveals massive accumulations of virus particles in the nuclei, bringing many of the nuclei to the point of rupture. Lesions are not found in trachea, heart, esophagus, brain, or kidney.

A presumptive diagnosis is based upon typical history and absence of other signs. Dead birds are well fleshed, but have the characteristic lesions of marble spleen and lung edema. Confirmation is based on serological tests and microscopic findings. Laboratory examination is done by the reverse agar gel precipitin (AGP) method, whereby splenic tissues of affected birds are reacted with positive pheasant or turkey serum. Or, the laboratory examination is done by the standard AGP in which serums from recovered pheasants are tested against marble spleen disease virus antigen.

TREATMENT AND CONTROL:

Provide clean fresh water and feed. Vaccinating with MSD vaccine via the drinking water will stop spread of the disease. Midtherapeutic levels of nitrofuran drugs and antibiotics will prevent secondary bacterial infections. Upgrade the quality of environment to enhance the comfort of the birds. Surviving birds appear to be immune.

Control measures are focused on containing the disease by pen — use quarantine, a separate caretaker, prevention of all cross traffic, prompt incineration of dead birds, and strict sanitation. Vaccinate birds in adjacent pens to prevent the spread of the disease.

PREVENTION:

Vaccinate young pheasants with commercial MSD vaccine. The MSD virus is used for turkeys. Low-pathogenic turkey HE virus is used to produce MSD vaccine. Pheasant chicks should be vaccinated via drinking water when 6 weeks of age. It is important that the vaccine be administered in water fountains that the pheasant chicks have been using. Pheasants will respond more uniformly if the young birds are vaccinated before being moved from the brooding to the growing pens. Recovered and/or vaccinated birds are immune to recurrent outbreaks. Growers are advised to vaccinate all subsequent hatches for at least 2 years. MSD can become repeatedly problematic on infected farms because the virus is persistent in the environment.

NEWCASTLE DISEASE

DEFINITION:

Newcastle Disease (ND) is an acute, rapidly spreading, contagious respiratory disease characterized by respiratory distress, encephalitis, or both. Synonyms are Newcastle, ND, and pneumoencephalitis. ND is caused by a paramyxovirus, Type I, that will agglutinate chicken RBC. It will grow in chicken embryos, and in a variety of chicken embryo tissue cell lines. Incubation requires from 5 to 7 days and the course of the disease is 10 to 14 days. The virus will survive in litter for 2 months and in infected dead birds for possibly 12 months. The virus is killed by disinfectants, fumigants, and direct sunlight. ND virus survives for only a short time in egg incubators. The three pathogenic types of virus endemic in the USA are lentogenic (mild field virus), mesogenic (intermediate virulence), and velogenic (extremely virulent). Virus pathotype or virulence is determined by severity of the disease.

All avian species of all ages are susceptible. The disease spreads across bird-species lines. Younger birds are more seriously affected. Morbidity is considered to be 100 percent but mortality is variable, depending on bird susceptibility and the pathotype of the ND virus involved. In pigeons, many surviving birds develop neurological signs. ND occurs in major poultry producing areas worldwide. In many countries a virulent fourth type of ND virus or viscerotropic velogenic ND (VVND) prevails. VVND does not yet exist in poultry-producing areas of the USA, but is common in pet caged birds smuggled into the country.

VVND is so virulent that it produces high mortality (usually 100%) in susceptible birds. Turkeys and peafowl are less susceptible than chickens. The turkey ND virus is classified as PMV-3.

TRANSMISSION AND CLINICAL SIGNS:

ND can be airborne. It can be transmitted on shoes of the caretaker, visitors, or service personnel, and on contaminated equipment. ND virus is passed through the egg, but infected embryos die before hatching. The virus lives for a short time in the incubator. Vertical transmission is not known to occur. Virus is shed during the clinical stage of the disease.

ND virus is present in exhaled air, respiratory exudates, feces, in eggs laid during the clinical phase, and all body tissues of dead birds. Turkeys and peafowl maintain a persistent ND viremia. The virus level in the blood correlates inversely with the antibody titer of the bird. As the antibody titer increases, the viremia level decreases. The circulating antibody level effectively eliminates the virus from the blood. Clinical signs are respiratory and/or nervous activity.

ND is usually of sudden onset, and may be accompanied by depression and anorexia. Baby birds show discomfort by huddling and chirping. Watery nasal discharges, labored breathing, trembling, paralysis, and twisting of the necks may appear. Neurological signs occur in a few birds, but such signs are more prevalent in nongallinaceous species.

The course of the disease within the flock is 10 to 14 days. Mortality in young susceptible birds ranges from 10 to 80 percent, depending on the virus pathotype invoved. In adult birds, symptoms include depression, loss of appetite, and severe drop in egg production. Production recovery usually takes 5 to 6 weeks which severely shortens the gamebird-breeding season. In terminal stages of ND birds have greenish diarrhea, facial swelling, clonic spasms, and other neurological signs.

LESIONS AND DIAGNOSIS:

Gross lesions may be minimal in young birds because of the acuteness of the disease. Death occurs before lesions can develop. All tissues are congested and hemorrhagic. Other lesions are facial swelling, cloudy air sacs, exudates in the lungs, trachea, and air sacs. Additional lesions are inflammation of all air passages from nares to air sacs and hemorrhagic, ruptured, and shriveled yolks in hens in production. Severity of lesions is related to the virus pathotype. The more virulent the field virus the more severe the lesions. VVND, exotic form, involves all the abdominal organs while endemic ND localizes in the respiratory and/or nervous systems. With the exotic form, hemorrhage at the stomach-gizzard junction is diagnostic. Velogenic ND kills the birds that have neurological lesions before the onset of respiratory signs. A clinical diagnosis can be made from history, signs, and lesions.

ND has been thoroughly researched. A variety of laboratory diagnostic procedures — including fluorescent antibody test, virus isolation, various serological tests, and HA tests on lung or other tissue fluids — are available. ND virus agglutinates chicken RBC, a feature in common with myxoviruses. The HA test is a valuable confirmatory test for suspect ND isolates or as a quick test on fresh respiratory fluids during diagnostic case work-up. Velogenic and VVND-suspect outbreaks are reportable to the State Veterinarian.

TREATMENT AND CONTROL:

There is no specific or helpful treatment for ND. The course of the disease is from 10 to 14 days. Most outbreaks are over by the time a laboratory confirmatory diagnosis is made. Supportive therapy, consisting of vitamins and/or a mid range dose of antibiotics, is recommended. To help young birds, make management adjustments such as raising room temperature and providing fresh feed and water to encourage eating and drinking. Promptly remove and incinerate dead birds.

DO NOT VACCINATE DURING AN OUTBREAK! Control is directed toward husbandry and management by doing things to contribute to the comfort of the birds. The VVND form of the disease is not endemic in the USA. As such, there are stringent federal laws regarding importing poultry, pet, and tropical caged birds. Because of the risk of VVND, it is poor judgment and practice for gamebird and poultry producers or their staff members to own or keep exotic and tropical pet caged birds. VVND outbreaks occur every year in this country in imported or smuggled pet caged birds. APHIS acts promptly and swiftly to eradicate each outbreak. VVND poses a severe health and economic threat to the entire gamebird and poultry industry of the USA. Economically, the presence of VVND in the US could double poultry production costs. To control outbreaks, exercise biosecurity and good husbandry measures to prevent spread of ND to other farms and to minimize mortality. Recovered birds are immune and do not shed the virus.

PREVENTION:

Prevention is accomplished by immunization and vigorous biosecurity (i.e., maximum effort to avoid the introduction of ND). Most gamebird producers do not vaccinate for ND until it becomes a problem on their farm or in their geographic area.

ND immunity is not life-long. Vaccinations are initiated while chicks are still in the brooder house. For breeders, revaccinate with live ND vaccines at 3-month intervals, with the breeder flock getting the last vaccination 30 days before the onset of production. ND vaccination can be done by spray, eye drop, or drinking water administration. Each procedure has specific DOs and DON'Ts designed to assure good immune response. If ND vaccination is needed or anticipated, consult a poultry veterinarian for a program for your farm and area.

PIGEON PARAMYXOVIRUS

DEFINITION:

Pigeon Paramyxovirus (PMV) infection is an acute infectious febrile disease of pigeons characterized by depression, loose droppings, neurological signs, and death. Other names are PMV, paramyxo, and parainfluenza. PMV is caused by a paramyxovirus. Incubation requires from 2 to 7 days and course of the disease is 10 to 14 days. Myxoviruses are named from the Greek *MYXO*, referring to nasal secretions or slime. PMV viruses include pigeon PMV and Newcastle disease (ND) of gamebirds, chickens, and wild song birds.

Most characteristics and properties of ND virus are shared by other paramyxoviruses. They are hemagglutination positive (HA), cross-reacting serologically, and growing in chicken embryos. PMV is immunologically distinct from influenza (orthomyxovirus), and antigenically stable, i.e., genetic recombination does not occur as it does in influenza viruses.

Pigeons of all ages are susceptible, but PMV is more serious in young birds. The virus will infect doves, chickens, and other avian hosts. There is no gender or breed difference. PMV occurs worldwide, wherever pigeons are kept. The disease may appear throughout the year, though in England most cases occur from August through October.

In the USA, outbreaks occur in Spring and Fall. The disease spreads during homing-pigeon trials; adult trials are held in the Spring and young pigeon trials in the Fall. Birds from all contestant hobbyists are shipped together to the release site. Exposure to subclinical carrier birds can occur during the transit period. Outbreaks occur in the various lofts after fliers return home.

TRANSMISSION AND CLINICAL SIGNS:

The virus is spread by contact between birds or exposure of birds to infective materials and premises, such as exudates, crates, lofts, or litter. Other opportunities for exposure occur during flight training, races, shows, and bird swaps. Experimentally infected pigeons excreted the virus from day 16 to day 31 following inoculation but showed no detectable antibodies until day 27. Chickens housed with infected pigeons shed virus in the droppings and became sero-positive, but showed no clinical signs. Ingestion and inhalation are the primary infection routes. The virus is excreted in the feces and exudates of infected pigeons.

Feral pigeons have been shown to harbor and to spread the virus to other pigeons and chickens. The virus is highly infectious to pigeons but it spreads slowly. Pigeons exposed to the LaSota strain of ND virus did not develop clinical signs but did so when inoculated with PMV virus. The duration varies with the virus strain and level of immunity from previous exposures, but becomes chronic within the loft.

Morbidity is from 20 to 80 percent and mortality may be as high as 90 percent. Infected birds have loose watery greenish droppings, depression, inappetence, weight loss, are reluctant to move, have ruffled feathers, are thirsty, and incoordinated. Infected birds have difficulty flying, walking, and eating. Wings and head tremble. There is partial paralysis of wings and legs and twisting of the neck. During the viremic stage, 2 to 3 weeks postinfection, pigeons become unwilling to fly.

LESIONS AND DIAGNOSIS:

There are no diagnostic lesions. Lesions and changes observed include hemorrhage of intestinal mucosa, cloaca, pancreas, and proventriculus. Congestion is present in lung, liver, spleen, kidney, and air sacs. Greenish discoloration of the liver, enteritis, and weight loss is also present.

A presumptive diagnosis is based on history, signs, and lesions. Most PMV cases have a history of one or more birds with twisted necks (i.e., neurological signs) that are indicative of the infection. Diagnostic confirmation is dependent on virus isolation and identification, microscopic demonstration of encephalitic lesions, and serological demonstration of humoral antibodies. The presence of antibodies confirms exposure to PMV and high titers are equated with immune responses resulting from a field outbreak. Birds with neurological signs are ruined as competitive homing pigeons.

PMV must be differentiated from influenza, herpes, ND, salmonella, and aspergillus infections.

TREATMENT AND CONTROL:

No specific treatment is effective. Adjust feed and water for easy access by sick and disoriented birds. Keep birds comfortable. It is not necessary to eliminate infected birds, but paralyzed birds should be culled. Recovered birds will be immune.

Control of PMV is directed toward disease prevention, focusing on biosecurity, isolation of newly purchased birds, close observation of birds after races, and application of good husbandry and sanitation practices.

PREVENTION:

A PMV vaccination program should be developed and closely followed by every racing-pigeon hobbyist. The PMV pigeon vaccine is an inactivated virus product that must be inoculated INTO EACH BIRD, either subcutaneously or intramuscularly. Inactivated vaccines do not spread, thus only inoculated birds will develop immunity.

Nonvaccinated birds remain susceptible and will become infected if exposed. Most vaccination programs recommend at least two inoculations at 30-day intervals. An annual booster should be administered 30 days before racing events or pairing for mating.

Some pigeon fanciers have used the live chicken ND vaccine. The hazard of this is the entire loft must be vaccinated at the same time, and many squabs and juvenile birds may be too young to safely vaccinate. The immune protection from live ND vaccines lasts between 90 and 120 days. The inactivated vaccine is safer and recommended. Follow instructions of manufacturer of vaccine for dose and method of administration.

QUAIL BRONCHITIS

DEFINITION:

Quail bronchitis is an acute, infectious, contagious, and highly fatal disease of bobwhite quail that affects birds in the wild and in captivity. QB is characterized by respiratory distress, catarrhal tracheitis, airsacculitis, and death. QB is the only synonym. The disease is caused by an adenovirus (type I, serotype I) and was originally called CELO for chick embryo lethal orphan that is widespread in chickens and several gamebird species. Turkeys can be infected experimentally.

The QB virus is isolated and propagated in chicken embryos or different tissue culture cell lines. Incubation requires 4 to 7 days and the disease runs its course in 3 to 5 weeks. Morbidity is 100 percent, and mortality commonly 50 percent. Quail and chickens are susceptible and considered to be natural hosts, with many chickens being inapparent carriers. Quail younger than 4 weeks are the most susceptible.

QB was first recognized in 1949 and is known to occur in quail throughout the USA. The disease is most prevalent in the southern states where there are many captive flocks of quail and large populations of quail thrive in the wild.

TRANSMISSION AND CLINICAL SIGNS:

The probable sources of QB are infected breeders (i.e., by transovarian passage), carrier birds, contaminated feces, or exudates brought onto the premises. Once introduced, the disease spreads rapidly by ingestion of infectious materials. QB is explosive and spreads rapidly through multi-age flocks on the farm. There is evidence that the disease is transmitted to quail by other bird species.

Clinical manifestations are respiratory distress with coughs, sneezes, rales, lacrimation, and conjunctivitis. Infected birds go off feed and water, chill, become weak and prostrate, and die. Subacutely affected birds develop a loose watery diarrhea.

Neurological signs occur in a few birds. The disease, most serious in birds younger than 4 weeks, is but mild or subclinical in birds older than 8 weeks. The course of QB in nontreated quail is 3 to 5 weeks; in chickens and turkeys it is 3 weeks. QB remains on the farm for the duration of the season, infecting each successive hatch.

LESIONS AND DIAGNOSIS:

Early lesions are excess mucus with roughness of the mucosa in the trachea and bronchi. Air sacs may be cloudy or thick. The QB virus also produces scattered pale whitish foci in the liver. The lungs are reddened with firm pneumonic lesions and the spleen is swollen and mottled. The trachea may contain free blood with opaque white areas on the mucosa.

Mucoid enteritis with gaseous distention of the intestine may be present. Dwarfing and deaths are seen in infected embryos during virus-isolation procedures. Histologically, there is a loss of cilia in the trachea and bronchi and hyperplasia of respiratory epithelium. Plaques of lymphocytes are seen in the propria layer of the trachea and bronchi. Intranuclear inclusions (viral clumps) are present in the respiratory epithelium. Liver and spleen lesions are similar to those of inclusion body hepatitis.

Other changes include histiocytic hyperplasia, fibrinoid necrosis, and depletion of lymphocytes. The bursa of Fabricius shows lymphoid depletion and atrophy. Viral inclusions are present in the mucosal epithelium. A presumptive diagnosis can be based on history, clinical signs, and lesions. Confirmation requires laboratory isolation of the virus, demonstration of bluish (basophilic) nuclear inclusions of respiratory epithelium, liver, bursa, and lymphoid depletion with hyperplasia of the spleen. The virus can be isolated in chicken embryos or chick embryo kidney cells. Serological tests are of limited value. The agar gel immunodiffusion (AGID) test will reveal the presence of antibodies to adenovirus serotype I.

TREATMENT AND CONTROL:

There is no specific treatment. Commercial vaccine is not available. Raise temperature in brooding houses 3 to 5° to prevent the birds from piling up and smothering. Other management adjustments include elimination of drafts, expansion of floor space per bird, adequate sanitation, and strict isolation and biosecurity. Avoid multiple-age operations and eliminate other stresses.

Antibiotics may provide control of opportunistic bacteria. Always provide fresh feed and water to encourage feeding and drinking. The disease will be perpetuated if new hatches of day-old quail are exposed or brooded near infected birds. Immunity is long-lasting, perhaps for life. Recovered birds should be retained as breeders because they are immune and provide maternal protection to progeny.

PREVENTION:

Break the cycle by depopulating, followed by thorough cleaning and disinfecting of pens and equipment. Follow C& D with a 30- to 90-day quarantine of facilities before repopulating. QB usually occurs during the hatching and growing season. Establish tight biosecurity to avoid exposing the new season's hatches.

Establish a vaccination program using an autogenous vaccine made from last year's virus isolates (a commercial vaccine is not available). Vaccination (Molthroup) program can be done as follows:

  i) Vaccinate breeders with autogenous vaccine by eye drop 8 weeks before onset of production.
  ii) Repeat 4 weeks later.
  iii) Chicks from immune breeders have a high parental immunity.
  iv) Hold vaccinated breeders in isolation to prevent spread of pathogens.

To prevent cross-exposure, use separate caretakers for breeders and chicks

ROTAVIRUS ENTERITIS

DEFINITION:

Rotavirus enteritis (RE) is a recognized enteric disease of several bird species. This disease is characterized by enteritis, diarrhea, dehydration, and stunting in young birds. The disease is referred to as RE, rotavirus, enterovirus, and runting disease. The causative agent is a rotavirus of which there are four distinct serological groups: **A, B, C,** and **D**. Group **A** rotavirus cross-reacts with mammalian rotavirus. Groups **B** and **C** have not been fully described. Group **D** rotaviruses have been found only in birds. Rotaviruses are double-stranded RNA viruses; replication occurs in the cytoplasm of the intestinal mucosal cells.

Presently, the Group **D** rotaviruses of different bird species are thought to be the same virus. Cross-infection between bird species occurs in 2 to 5 days postinfection. Incubation requires 2 to 5 days and the course of the disease is 3 to 4 weeks. Pheasants, ducks, turkeys, chickens, pigeons, Guinea fowl, and love birds are known to be susceptible to rotavirus. Young birds are the most susceptible. Current reports indicate that rotaviruses have worldwide distribution. Much of the research on avian rotaviruses was done in European and Asian countries.

TRANSMISSION AND CLINICAL SIGNS:

Transmission is horizontal by the oral route. Egg passage has not been demonstrated. Rotaviruses are excreted in large numbers in the feces. No data on the fate of the virus in the feces are available, but from observation, environmental contamination is persistent. Successive birds break with the disease when placed on the infected litter. Cleaning and disinfecting is the only effective method to break the cycle within the rearing facility. The infection readily spreads from bird to bird. Rotavirus has been found in 3-day-old poults.

There is no evidence that recovered birds remain carriers. In broilers, clinical signs varied from subclinical to severe, with diarrhea associated with dehydration, poor weight gains, and increased mortality. Early clinical signs are diarrhea (wet litter), depression, and poor appetite within 2 to 5 days following infection. Dehydration occurs rapidly and mortality increases to 30 to 50 percent in pheasants and turkeys. Survivors appear healthy but stunted or smaller. Delayed or recurrent infections characterized by restlessness, eating of litter, watery droppings, and mortality up to 7 percent have been reported in poults 12 to 21 days of age. Mortality is much higher in younger birds; they chill, pile up, and suffocate. Rotavirus can be demonstrated in droppings randomly selected from the flock experiencing an outbreak.

Susceptible adult birds experience outbreaks. It is thought that most older birds become exposed to and develop immunity to the rotavirus before reaching maturity. Adult birds have diarrhea associated with the rotavirus infection.

LESIONS AND DIAGNOSIS:

The most common finding on necropsy is abnormal amounts of fluid and gas in the intestine and ceca. Other findings include dehydration, inflamed vents, anemia, litter in the gizzard, and inflammation and fecal encrustation on the foot pads.

Microscopically, the villi of the intestinal mucosa are shortened. Each rotavirus group tends to prefer a specific area of the intestine. Group A rotavirus concentrates in the duodenum while Group D rotavirus is found in the jejunum. Histological changes are villus atrophy, thickening of the lamina propria, scalloping of the villus surface, fusion of villi, and leukocytic infiltration. Villi become shortened and crypts become deeper. No immunofluorescence is observed in the proventriculus, gizzard, spleen, liver, and kidney.

Diagnosis requires the isolation and identification of the pathogen. Electron microscopy (EM) demonstration of rotavirus in fecal material of sick birds is the most common laboratory procedure. EM is sensitive enough and detects rotaviruses of all serogroups.

Virus isolation is not a satisfactory procedure for avian rotaviruses. Virus isolation by tissue culture is useful only for the Group A rotaviruses. Serological procedures are not reliable because specific reagents are not commercially available. Immunofluorescent staining is used to demonstrate the virus in infected feces or intestinal contents. Immunofluorescent staining and EM are the most reliable laboratory diagnostic procedures for this disease. Rotavirus must be differentiated from other intestinal infections.

TREATMENT AND CONTROL:

At present there is no specific treatment or means of controlling rotavirus enteritis. Rotavirus is ubiquitous, and it is not practical to try to keep commercial flocks free of infection. Commercial vaccines are not available.

The effect of diarrhea on the litter (i.e., as the infection source) can be minimized by increasing ventilation and by adding fresh litter. If fresh litter is not used, diseases and health problems become more severe with each successive flock.

The usual procedure to breaking the cycle of rotavirus infections in a facility is depopulation, thorough C& D, and resting the premises (i.e., leaving them empty) for up to 4 weeks. Birds for repopulating must come from a source known to be free of the disease. Since rotavirus is not transmitted THROUGH THE EGG, chicks from the resident breeder flock should be used. Precautions would focus on egg and hatchery sanitation, prevention of cross-traffic in the hatchery, and biosecurity for the premises.

The above measures are recommended for diseases that cannot be controlled or prevented by other strategies, e.g., medication, vaccination, or isolation.

PREVENTION:

Prevention of rotavirus infections relies upon good overall management, including farm-wide biosecurity, all-in all-out bird production, and daily pen sanitation. Remove and dispose of dead birds promptly.

Procure chicks from disease-free sources. Provide a balanced diet, appropriate preventive medication, and a health program designed for the farm. Experimentally, live attenuated rotavirus given in the drinking water have been more effective than injections of inactivated autogenous vaccines. The live vaccine should be used in breeder-replacement birds 30 to 60 days before the onset of production. Progeny has maternal immunity from experimental breeder vaccination. Growers are advised to get a laboratory diagnosis early in the outbreak of the disease. Once rotavirus is confirmed, control and preventive measures should be initiated promptly.

TRANSMISSIBLE ENTERITIS

DEFINITION:

Transmissible enteritis is an acute, infectious, contagious disease of turkeys of all ages that is characterized by depression, low body temperature, loss of appetite, loss of weight, watery feces, prostration, and death. The disease is also known as mud fever, bluecomb, TE, coronaviral enteritis, CE, and infectious enteritis.

TE is caused by a coronavirus but clinically the disease is complicated by other viral and bacterial infections of the intestine. Incubation requires 48 to 72 hours and the course of the disease is 10 to 14 days. The virus has not been adapted to tissue culture but can be grown in 15-day-old turkey embryos. The virus localizes in the intestine and bursa of Fabricius of young poults. The virus remains pathogenic after 110 turkey embryo passages. The disease is not related to "bluecomb" of chickens or hemorrhagic enteritis of turkeys. The virus appears to be resistant in the turkey-house environment. Experimentally, the virus was easily destroyed in batteries and cages but survived well in frozen feces. Freezing weather increases survival of the virus.

Under field conditions, eradication requires depopulating, thorough C& D, and resting of pens for 3 to 4 weeks. Susceptibility of birds is influenced by age and environmental conditions; mortality in young flocks can be as high as 50 percent. Chickens, pheasant, sea gulls, and coturnix quail were resistant to experimental infections.

TRANSMISSION AND CLINICAL SIGNS:

TE spreads by contact with infected birds or contaminated premises. Feces of infected birds are rich in virus. Recovered birds remain carriers and virus shedders for several months, perhaps for life. Once in the flock, TE spreads rapidly. Natural outbreaks are the result of ingesting infectious materials.

Stress and adverse environmental conditions contribute to the severity of the disease. Experimentally, TE is transmitted by intestinal material given by the oral or rectal routes. Suspensions of heart, liver, spleen, and kidney did not infect day-old poults. Filtrates from the bursa of Fabricius given by mouth did infect poults. Bursal filtrates were pathogenic even to adult turkeys.

TE spreads to other farms via personnel, equipment and vehicles, and free-flying birds. Early clinical signs are sudden onset and rapid spread. The incubation period of 2 to 3 days is followed by depression, anorexia, and diarrhea. Young poults chill, chirp constantly, and seek heat. Feed and water consumption drops severely and poults lose weight rapidly. In untreated outbreaks, morbidity and mortality may reach 100 percent . As the disease progresses, feces show mucus threads with urates and may be green from bile stains.

Symptoms are similar, but less severe, in adult turkeys. Egg production decreases and some egg shells will be chalky. The clinical course of the disease is 10 to 14 days. Birds require several weeks to regain weight. Mature males never fully regain lost weight, producing an obvious unevenness of size within the flock.

LESIONS AND DIAGNOSIS:

There is dehydration, cyanosis of the head, and emaciation of ill turkeys. Gross lesions are seen in the intestine as catarrhal enteritis and flaccid intestinal walls with bulbous areas. In some birds, the intestinal contents are watery with excess mucus and protein casts. The pancreas has a white chalky appearance; kidneys and ureters are distended with urates; and the spleen is shrunken, pale, and gray. The crop may be swollen and its contents soured.

Microscopically, the intestinal changes are shortened villi, loss of goblet cells, and separation of mucosa from the intestinal wall. Other changes include urate nephritis, large numbers of round cells in the adrenal glands, and focal hydropic pancreatic degeneration with eosinophilic intracytoplasmic inclusions.

A presumptive diagnosis is based on history of the outbreak, clinical signs, gross lesions, and absence of other causes (e.g., bacteria and protozoa). Laboratory confirmation requires one or more techniques — such as FA, detection of coronavirus in the intestinal contents by electron microscopy (EM), and reproducing the disease in SPF poults with bacteria-free intestinal filtrates. The direct fluorescent antibody (FA) model can be used to identify the virus in intestinal epithelium, cecum, or bursa of Fabricius. Indirect FA can be used as serological test to detect antibodies in convalescent serum. TE must be differentiated from other enteric diseases such as hexamitiasis, paratyphoid, and rotaviral infections.

TREATMENT AND CONTROL:

Antibiotics may suppress mortality. Medicate the feed with antibiotics for one week, then administer vitamins with electrolytes in the drinking water intermittently for 3 days per period. After 14 days, harvest blood samples from 20 poults for serological tests.

Empirical therapy includes a dairy-calf milk replacer [25 lb/100 gal] or potassium chloride [1 lb/100 gal] in drinking water for 3 days. For adult turkeys, add molasses [1 pint/5 gal] drinking water for 1 day to flush the birds before begining antibiotic therapy. Control depends on management and improved sanitation that contributes to the comfort and well being of the birds. Younger birds require additional heat. During and following treatment, observe birds closely for secondary intestinal mycosis, a condition often following a heavy regimen of antibiotics.

PREVENTION:

Eradicate TE on the outbreak farm by the usual procedures of de-population and C&D. Leave the premises empty for 4 weeks. Re-populate with birds from TE-free sources. Recovered birds are carriers and virus shedders for long periods, perhaps for life. Development of a safe effective vaccine is currently unlikely due to the inability to at-tenuate the coronavirus.

An alternative to TE eradication is the establishment of a "Controlled Exposure" program. Such a program is not without its problems. Pro-ducers should seek advice from state officials, producer organizations, and nearby producers before deciding on this approach. "Controlled Exposure" should be considered only in unusual circumstances. Eradication should always be the first approach to the prevention of TE.

GROWER'S REFERENCE

ON

GAMEBIRD HEALTH

IV. PROTOZOAN DISEASES — 153

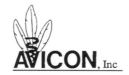

AVICON, Inc

COCCIDIOSIS

DEFINITION:

Avian coccidiosis is a disease caused by a protozoan parasite. The disease is characterized by enteritis and diarrhea and is of universal importance in the production of gamebirds and poultry. Avian coccidia are host- (i.e., species-) and site-specific, i.e., they infect the intestinal tract. An exception is *Eimeria truncata,* a renal coccidiosis that infects the kidneys of geese and swans. Even subclinical coccidiosis, i.e., infection without clinical signs, causes economic losses. Coxy or cocci are the common synonyms for the disease.

Coccidia are single-celled parasitic protozoan organisms of the sporozoan group that belongs to the genus Eimeria. Eimeria oocysts (eggs) contain four sporocysts. Each sporocyst contains two sporozoites (infective units), thus eight infective units occupy each oocyst.

Multiple coccidia species infect each bird species. Avian coccidia are host-specific and will not cross-infect other species of birds, for example, coccidia that infect quail will not infect chukar or pheasants. The reverse is true. There are at least four species of coccidia that infect pheasants and at least four species can be found in quail, chukar, etc. There are nine coccidial species of chickens and eight species in wild and domestic turkeys. Coccidiosis is largely a disease of young birds because immunity develops after exposure. There is no cross-immunity between species of coccidia.

Subsequent outbreaks will occur when birds are exposed to a different species of coccidia. Immunity is short-lived unless birds are in continual contact with coccidia. Coccidiosis may strike any type of poultry in any type of facility. Most avian brooding and rearing pens offer ideal environmental conditions (i.e., heat, humidity, and moist litter) for rapid growth and replication of coccidia. Coccidia have a short direct life cycle and high reproductive potential. The life cycle is from 7 to 9 days, during which there are eight developmental stages. The oocysts sporulate in litter within 36 to 48 hours. Once sporulated, they are infective. Coccidiosis is a worldwide avian disease common in pen-raised pheasant, quail, chukar, turkeys, chickens, pigeons, Guinea fowl, ducks, and geese. Every gamebird producer must develop a coccidiosis control program.

TRANSMISSION AND CLINICAL SIGNS:

Coccidiosis is borne on litter and fecal material. Birds become infected by swallowing feces, infected litter, or contaminated feed or water. Infection occurs only if the bird ingests infective oocysts. Coxy does not spread directly from bird to bird. It spreads indirectly from oocysts in the litter to susceptible birds. Oocysts are present on floors, in litter, or in soil of pens previously occupied by infected birds.

Oocysts are easily transported to other premises by people, vehicles, and equipment. People are important vectors. Clinical signs vary with the pathogenicity of the infecting coccidia. Weakness, paleness, ruffled feathers, general unthriftiness, diarrhea, and death are common outward signs of coccidiosis outbreaks. Droppings may be bloody but more often are whitish and semisolid in texture. Affected birds show depression, sit around, and have little interest in feed or water. Mortality can be high and is related to the coccidia species involved, and to the pen conditions that triggered the outbreak. Coccidia need moisture to sporulate; therefore, outbreaks occur when susceptible birds are put into infected pens or when litter becomes wet and the temperature is warm. In poorly drained outdoor pens in wet seasons, similar conditions cause coccidiosis outbreaks.

Recovered birds develop immunity to coccidia, but this protection can be overwhelmed if massive numbers of infective oocysts are ingested, as would be the case with wet litter or wet outdoor pens. Accumulated mortality can be high if treatment or control measures are delayed or withheld. Mild infections may cause depigmentation of skin and legs. Survivors recover in 10 to 14 days.

LESIONS AND DIAGNOSIS:

Except for renal coccidiosis of geese, all coccidia of gamebirds and domestic poultry are confined to intestines and ceca. Primary coccidial lesions are ballooning of the intestine with fetid odor; enteritis, intestinal or cecal core; speckled appearance of serosal surface of intestine; and creamy catarrhal intestinal contents. Whitish foci on the serosal intestinal wall are evidence of the presence of colonies of coccidia. Coccidia may cause pin-point hemorrhages on the outer wall of the intestine; these colonies plus the hemorrhages create the speckled appearance.

Each coccidia species has a preferred region of the intestine where it resides (upper, middle, or lower). In most field breaks, multiple species are present, and they may cause lesions the full length of intestine. Speciating the coccidia in an outbreak is not needed. A diagnosis of coccidiosis can be based on flock history, signs, and intestinal lesions. Microscopic demonstration of oocysts in feces or intestinal scrapings confirms the diagnosis. The presence of oocysts alone can be an accurate confirmation.

Other factors, such as flock appearance and performance, morbidity, mortality, number of birds having intestinal lesions, and intestinal odor are important in assessing the severity of the outbreak. Most experienced gamebird producers readily recognize typical intestinal lesions caused by coccidia. Most laboratory reports will list the diagnosis as "Intestinal coccidiosis," meaning that more than one coccidial species is present.

TREATMENT AND CONTROL:

All sulfa drugs are active against coccidia but they vary in toxicity to birds. Sulfadimethoxine (SDM), a newer, safer drug, is usually prescribed. Sulfaquinoxaline (SQ) and sulfamethazine, older drugs, are effective, but more toxic. These older drugs should never be administered for more than 3 consecutive days. SDM is safe for up to 7 days of continuous administration. Amprolium, a coccidiostat, is safe for use in drinking water.

Outbreak treatment must be fast and effective, and thus requires medication by drinking water. Most growers routinely use a coccidiostat in the feed, but outbreaks occur in spite of this medication.

To avoid drug toxicity in such cases, flock medication during outbreaks should employ a drug different from that routinely fed in the feed. For example, if continuous Amprolium medication is used in the feed, treat outbreaks with SDM in the water or visa versa.

Controlling coccidiosis outbreaks requires immediate medication to avoid further mortality, followed by management action to correct the environment. Replace wet litter and increase room ventilation to dry the remaining litter. After mortality stops, add vitamins and electrolytes to the water for 2 to 3 days. This will hasten recovery.

Coccidial infections cause severe tissue damage to the intestinal mucosa, leading to anemia by loss of blood. Vitamins and electrolytes contribute to tissue repair and blood formation. Check feed for presence and level of coccidiostat and make adjustments accordingly.

PREVENTION:

Sanitation, plus a coccidiostat in the feed, is the best method of preventing coccidiosis. Management factors include good dry litter at all times and changing litter after each flock. Proper ventilation helps to keep litter dry as the moving air exhausts warm air and carries away excess moisture from the pens. Litter of proper moisture content will almost hold its shape when squeezed by hand.

The litter will become dusty with less moisture and more damp with more moisture. Coccidia need moisture to sporulate, thus by keeping the litter dry, flock managers can prevent coccidiosis. Be aware of wet spots around waterers or damp litter when birds have diarrhea. Keep the flock healthy from other infections to prevent situations that lead to coccidiosis.

In summary, use coccidiostats in the feed, keep litter dry by replacement and ventilation, and treat flock promptly for diarrhea.

COCCIDIOSTATS CLEARED BY F.D.A.

PRODUCT	CHEMICAL NAME	MANUFACTURER
Amprol	Amprolium	Merck (MSD AGVET)
Amprol-E	Amprolium + ethopabate	Merck (MSD AGVET)
Avatec	Lasalocid	Hoffman LaRoche
BioCox	Salinomycin	Agri Bio Corp
Bonaid	Buquinolate	Norwich Eaton
Coban (see below)	Monensin sodium	Elanco
Coyden-25	Clopidol - 25%	A.L. Laboratories
Deccox	Decoquinate	Rhone-Poulenc, Inc
Nicarb	Nicarbazin	Merck (MSD AGVET)
Rofenaid	Sulfadimethoxine, Ormetroprim	Hoffman LaRoche
Robenz	Robenidine HCL	American Cyanamid
Stenerol	Halofuginone Hydrobromide	Hoeschst-Roussel
SQ	Sulfaquinoxaline	Merck (MSD AGVET)
Zoamix	Zoalene	Solvay

These drugs are cleared for use in chicken and turkeys. Many are safe and effective for gamebirds too. Gamebird species vary in their drug susceptibility. A given coccidiostat may not be safe for all gamebird species.

Coban [73 g/ton] is FDA approved FOR QUAIL ONLY.

CRYPTOSPORIDIA

DEFINITION:

Cryptosporidiosis is a parasitic disease of birds. It is caused by a protozoan organism, and is characterized by acute and/or chronic infection of the respiratory and digestive tracts. The common reference is crypto. The causative organism is a coccidian protozoan of the genus cryptosporidium of which there are three known species affecting birds — *Cryptosporidium baileyi, C. meleagridis* , and one (unnamed) in quail. Quail, pheasant, peafowl, waterfowl, chickens, turkeys, finches, and psittacines are susceptible. Humans, other mammals, reptiles, amphibians, and fish are also susceptible. Some infections are asymptomatic.

The life cycle is similar to other coccidia involving asexual and sexual phases, replicating in the microvillus border of epithelial cells, and culminating in oocyst production. *C. baileyi* is believed to cause infections in the respiratory tract, cloaca, and bursa of Fabricius. *C. meleagridis* causes infection of the small intestine, especially of turkey and quail. The disease is usually fatal to quail and more serious in turkeys than in chickens. The susceptibility in other avian species has not been defined. Infective oocysts contain four naked sporozoites. In other coccidia, the sporozoite is contained in sporocysts within the oocyst. The life cycle is short (4 to 7 days) and the endogenous stages are small (4 to 7 mµ). The oocyst is very small, measuring 5 mµ. No known public health threat exists with avian cryptosporidia. Cryptosporidium appear to be present wherever birds are produced; therefore it can be found throughout the world.

TRANSMISSION AND CLINICAL SIGNS:

Transmission occurs when susceptible birds swallow infective oocysts. The oocysts, very resistant in the environment, are excreted in the feces of infected or carrier birds. The contamination of litter and soil provides a source of the infection in successive flocks. During the acute stage, very high numbers of oocysts are shed. Pen-to-pen and farm-to-farm spread of the disease is by transfer of oocysts on shoes, clothing, equipment, and people. The course of the disease is about 14 days. Immunity develops in 14 to 16 days, after which there is rapid clearance of the parasite.

In quail, respiratory and intestinal forms of cryptosporidia have both been reported. Clinical signs of the respiratory form include naso-ocular discharge, swollen sinuses, coughing, sneezing, dyspnea, and rales. Clinical signs of the intestinal form include diarrhea (often fatal in young turkeys, quail, and psittacines.) Mortality in young quail may reach 95 percent. Infected birds are depressed, have ruffled feathers, lose weight, sit in humped position, and may have soiled vent feathers. Litter may be damp because of the diarrhea.

LESIONS AND DIAGNOSIS:

Respiratory cryptosporidiosis causes mucoid exudates, either gray or white, on infected surfaces. Tissues affected in the respiratory form are conjunctiva, sinuses, nasal turbinates, lungs (they become gray), bronchi, and air sacs. Signs begin to appear in one week after exposure. Severe sinusitis develops in turkeys. Pulmonary infections show gray firm lungs. Intestinal lesions cause the gut to dilate with fluid. The ceca may be distended with foamy contents.

Histologic lesions include shortened villi, necrosis, loss of enterocytes from the villi tips, and presence of numerous cryptosporidia in brush borders of the intestinal mucosal epithelium. Cryptosporidia can be demonstrated in the cecal tonsil, in mucosa of the bursa of Fabricius, and in the cloaca. The bursal epithelium may be hyperplastic. Acute infections can be diagnosed by presence of oocysts in fresh feces or in fluids or scrapings of the respiratory tract. The organisms are basophilic with H&E stain, measure 2 to 4 μ in diameter, and found in the brush border of mucosal cells.

Laboratory procedures for identification of cryptosporidia are by bright-field or with phase-contrast microscopy, acid-fast staining, and negative staining with FA microscope. Collect specimens on moist cotton swabs. Vigorous swabbing of mucosa will collect oocysts from the epithelial border. Histological examination should be done on several sections of various organs.

Touch impressions can be examined by phase-contrast microscopy. Flotation techniques on feces include sucrose solution, saturated zinc sulfate, and sodium chloride. Oocysts are 4 μ in diameter and have a thick wall, prominent residual body, small dense bodies, and curved sporozoites. Other concurrent infections include candidiasis, paratyphoid, reovirus, and flagellated protozoa.

TREATMENT AND CONTROL:

All known anticoccidial drugs are ineffective against cryptosporidia. The macrolide antibiotic, spiramycin, is the only drug tested that has shown efficacy for treating *C. parvum* in humans. For birds, supportive therapy is recommended and could be beneficial in reducing mortality in concurrent infections. The younger the birds at onset, the greater the mortality from cryptsporidia. Control of outbreaks is focused on hygiene, sanitation, and biosecurity. Every management effort should be made to minimize the spread.

Cryptosporidia are resistant to germicides that kill bacterial, fungal, and viral pathogens. The use of the steam cleaner may be more effective and a safer means of disinfecting the floors and cages. Temperatures hotter than 65°C will kill the oocysts. Chemical germicides should be used when steam cleaning is not available. If the outbreak is confined to one flock with high mortality, it is advisable to destroy and incinerate the remainder of flock. Clean and steam treat the floors and equipment rather than risk the spread to adjacent pens or new bird placements. Throughout the outbreak, all birds removed should be incinerated.

PREVENTION:

Prevention of cryptosporidiosis is through biosecurity, good husbandry, and sanitary practices. There is no effective anticryptosporidia drug for treatment or prevention. Prevention for succeeding years may require depopulation and C&D (including steam-treatment of floors and equipment) of the premises 60 to 90 days before the new season begins. Rest the clean empty building for at least 60 days. Repopulate with day-old chicks (adult birds could reintroduce the disease.)

Cryptosporidiosis is not egg passed. If resident breeders are to be used, isolate the breeders from grow-out facilities. Use separate caretakers to avoid risk of infection from crosstraffic between pens of adult and young birds. Apply strict biosecurity measures within the operation and with all personnel.

HAEMOPROTEUS INFECTIONS

DEFINITION:

Haemoproteus is a malaria-like disease of pigeons and other avian species. Synonym is pigeon malaria. The disease is caused by protozoan organisms of the genus Haemoproteus. More than 120 species of haemoproteus exist and most are in wild birds — waterfowl, raptors, passerines, and other field birds. Like other protozoan blood parasites, (for example, leucocytozoa), haemoprotei are generally host-specific. In the asexual stage, haemoprotei are found in RBC rather than in white blood cells. Gametocytes (the mature sexual stage) contain a malarial pigment not present in leucocytozoa.

The parasite is essentially host-specific for the primary host, but can be spread by different intermediate hosts. *H. columbae* infects pigeons and doves; *H. nettionis* infects waterfowl; and *H. lophorytx* infects quail. Schizogony (i.e., asexual reproduction) occurs in the endothelial cells of internal organs rather than in the RBC as with Plasmodium, the cause of true malaria. Pigeons, doves, quail, ducks, turkeys, songbirds, and reptiles are susceptible. Pigeons are the most seriously affected bird species followed by muscovy ducks. A 1936 study identified infected birds of 45 wild species including owls, woodpeckers, and chipping sparrows. Infection in mammals has not been reported. Haemoproteus is widely distributed in tropical and temperate climates where the transmitting vector prevails year round. In cooler climates, the infection is sporadic and prevalent only during insect seasons. The disease has been reported in most of the USA, England, and tropical countries.

TRANSMISSION AND CLINICAL SIGNS:

This pathogen is transmitted by blood-sucking insects like other malaria or malaria-like protozoa. Culicoides, biting midges, transmit the disease to ducks but members of the fly genus Lynchia are vectors to other wild and domestic birds. Acutely affected birds exhibit signs similar to leucocytozoonosis or malaria. The onset is sudden with generalized weakness due to anemia. Birds are lethargic with loss of appetite. However, this parasite is not always a severe pathogen because it is known that many normal-appearing birds may harbor considerable numbers of the organism. Labored breathing, lameness, and death are observed in acute outbreaks.

LESIONS AND DIAGNOSIS:

The predominant lesion is anemia, as reflected by loss of RBC. Other lesions are engorgement of visceral vessels and swelling of the liver and spleen. During the acute phase, the liver and spleen are enlarged and dark, the heart is hemorrhagic, and the lungs are edematous. In muscovy ducks, the kidneys as well as the liver are swollen and firm. The diagnosis is based on history, signs, typical lesions, parasitized RBC on stained blood smears, and positive microscopic findings. There is an absence of other visible lesions. Blood smears and frozen tissue sections should be stained with Wright's or Giemsa stain.

TREATMENT AND CONTROL:

Medicate flock with antimalarial drugs such as quinacrine (Atabrine), primaquine, quinine, clopidol, or newer remedies as they become available. Always check the legality of the treatment suggested and comply with the withdrawal time for the drug used. Check warnings on label regarding safety of drug for birds to be medicated (some drugs may be toxic to certain species of birds). For example, arsenic or drugs containing arsenicals are extremely toxic to waterfowl.

PREVENTION:

Management, insect control, and low-level continuous medication provides the best method of prevention. However, prevention may not be possible in areas with populations of infected transmitter insects.

HEXAMITIASIS

DEFINITION:

Hexamitiasis is an acute disease of turkeys, pheasant, chukar, quail, pigeon, doves, and peafowl. The disease characterized by catarrhal enteritis with foamy, watery diarrhea. The synonym is infectious catarrhal enteritis. The causative agent is the protozoan *Hexamita meleagridis* in gallinaceous birds and *H. columbae* in pigeons and doves. The organism is 3 to 9 µ in length, has flagella and two nuclei, said to resemble eyes. The Hexamita organism moves rapidly with darting motions.

Birds of all susceptible species are vulnerable to the disease when younger than 9 weeks. Greatest losses occur between the ages of 3 and 8 weeks. Turkey poults develop resistance within 10 to 12 weeks of age. The disease is rarely found in adult birds. Chickens are not susceptible but may be inapparent carriers.

Hexamitiasis has been reported in many countries, including the United States. The disease usually occurs during the warmer months, thus correlating with the season of heaviest production. Poor sanitation in bird quarters adds to the severity of the disease.

TRANSMISSION AND CLINICAL SIGNS:

Transmission occurs from bird-to-bird contact and from ingestion of droppings or contaminated feed and water. Recovered birds are carriers and shed the parasite in their feces. Contamination of feed, water, litter, or range then occurs. Inter-species transmission from bird species to species occurs readily. Commingling of species in outdoor pens is thought to be a common avenue of spread.

Incidence of hexamitiasis will increase during the season when successive hatches are placed in infected pens. Morbidity is high and mortality may reach 75 to 90 percent in young untreated birds in unsanitary pens. Recovered carrier birds are often the source of new infections. Clinically affected poults and gamebirds show nervousness, chilling (they huddle around heat), have ruffled feathers, stilted gait, and watery or foamy diarrhea. Infected birds dehydrate rapidly. They continue to eat, but lose weight. Later the birds become depressed and listless, stand with heads retracted, feathers dull and ruffled, and wings droopy.

Terminal signs may be the result of electrolyte loss. Birds become comatose and recumbent, then die. Survivors are stunted and unthrifty, and otherwise poor in quality. Mortality tends to be highest in multi-aged flocks.

LESIONS AND DIAGNOSIS:

The cadaver is dehydrated, emaciated, and tissues are cyanotic. The intestines tend to be flabby with bulbous dilatations that contain excessive mucus, gas, and foamy material. The upper half of the intestine is inflamed and the cecal tonsils may be congested. The presence of watery diarrhea and demonstration of the organism in smears from fresh duodenum contents are sufficient evidence for diagnosis.

The organism is easily demonstrated with reduced-light or phase-contrast microscopy. Numerous hexamita in the upper intestine suggest hexamitiasis even though there may be no other lesions. The organism dies soon after the bird dies, therefore freshly expired birds or birds killed for necropsy offer the best chance of demonstrating the hexamita. If only recently expired birds are available, the organism may perhaps be revived by putting intestinal scrapings in a drop of warm saline solution on the slide. It is preferable to have live birds for necropsy. Finding a few hexamita in birds older than 10 weeks is not not considered supportive of diagnosis.

H. meleagridis is found in myriad numbers in intestinal crypts (Lieberkuhn); the organism attaches to the epithelial cells by its posterior flagella. Hexamitiasis must be differentiated from trichomoniasis, histomoniasis, paratyphoid, and viral enteric infections.

TREATMENT AND CONTROL:

Blackhead medications are effective against hexamitiasis. The nitrofurans and tetracyclines are likewise beneficial. Effectiveness of medication will be limited unless accompanied by improvements in husbandry and environment. Medication is no substitute for adequate sanitation and management. Sanitation is essential in all phases of bird care for control of hexamitiasis. During treatment, the brooder room temperature should be adjusted to the comfort of the birds. Administration of vitamins and electrolytes is good supplemental recovery therapy.

PREVENTION:

Prevention is accomplished by adopting practices implied by biosecurity and disease eradication. Short periods of depopulation combined with C&D of buildings will greatly reduce the population of Hexamita. Establish an all-in, all-out brooding and growing program with vigorous C& D between flocks. Placing new hatches in infected pens guarantees infection.

Clean and disinfect waterers daily and keep them on large wire platforms. Do not save birds from infected flocks for breeders. Raise only birds of the same age together. Have separate caretakers for young and adult birds. Minimize cross-traffic between flocks of different ages. Do not visit other farms. Keep visitors out of the pens.

HISTOMONIASIS

DEFINITION:

Histomoniasis is a protozoan disease of gamebirds, poultry, and gallinaceous birds. The disease is characterized by necrotizing lesions of the ceca and liver. Synonyms are blackhead and enterohepatitis, the latter describing the organs affected. The etiology is a protozoan parasite *Histomonas meleagridis.* *E.coli* and other coliform bacteria work synergistically with the histomonad to produce typical blackhead lesions.

H. meleagridis, while in the intestinal tract of birds, is an intestinal flagellate that assumes an ameboid form in the tissues. The protozoan in its nonameboid state is spherical and 3 to 16 mμ in size. A larger nonpathogenic four-flagellated histomonad, *H. wenrichi,* is found in the ceca. The cecal worm *Heterakis gallinarum* serves as the mechanical vector for *H. meleagridis.* Free living forms do not survive long, but the protozoan is quite resistant while inside the Heterakis egg or encysted in the earthworm. Three species of earthworms can harbor the infective heterakis egg or histomonad. Chukar, grouse, quail, partridge, pheasant, turkeys, and peafowl are quite susceptible but any avian specie under conducive circumstances can break with blackhead.

Chickens are often inapparent carriers and shedders of histomoniasis. Benefits of segregatiing birds (by species as well as by age) as a disease-control measure are well-documented. Birds younger than 12 weeks are the most susceptible to histomoniasis; turkeys are the most susceptible of the domestic poultry species. Histomoniasis historically is a serious disease consideration for birds growing on range, especially turkeys.

Of the gamebird species, chukar partridge appears to be the most susceptible to histomoniasis. The disease is widespread in the United States, especially in turkey- and gamebird-producing areas, and is present to a lesser extent in other countries. Histomoniasis is less troublesome for birds in confinement or reared on dry sandy ranges free of earthworms.

TRANSMISSION AND CLINICAL SIGNS:

The protozoan, many within the eggs of the cecal worm, is passed in the droppings of infected birds. Transmission of *H. meleagridis* to susceptible birds occurs when they ingest infected fresh feces, infective embryonated worm eggs, or earthworms containing the encysted worm larvae. Ingestion is the only route of transmission. The protozoan is very resistant when inside the worm eggs or in the earthworm and it is in this form that it is perpetuated on contaminated premises. Infected earthworms that survive the winter introduce the disease to susceptible birds the following spring.

Histomonads are released from Heterakis larvae in the ceca a few days after entry of the nematode. Histomanads reproduce rapidly in cecal tissues. The protozoan migrates into the deeper layers of the intestinal wall and causes inflammation and necrosis. Histomonads migrate to the liver via the blood stream or through the peritoneal cavity.

Round necrotic lesions quickly appear in the liver. Clinical signs appear within 7 to 12 days of exposure. Early signs include thirst, decreased appetite, watery yellow droppings, drowsiness, and weakness. As the disease progresses, birds develop dry ruffled feathers, become dehydrated, and lose weight. Tissues are dark or cyanotic. Birds stand with head drawn close to the body. Morbidity and mortality increase significantly. Death may reach 100 percent in untreated flocks. Young birds may die within a few days but older birds may linger, becoming emaciated by time of death.

LESIONS AND DIAGNOSIS:

Typical well-developed lesions are diagnostic. Experienced gamebird producers readily recognize lesions of histomoniasis. Most lesions are confined to the lower intestine, ceca, and liver. Caseous cores develop in the intestine and ceca. Cecal lesions show inflammatory changes and ulcerations, with a thickening of the wall. The core is yellow, gray, or green, and may be layered. The core develops from necrotic debris which includes exudates, tissue cells, pus cells, and the organisms. Peritonitis develops as the inflammation extends through the intestinal wall and is marked by a sticky texture and fetid odor.

Liver lesions are circular with depressed crater-like centers that vary in color from yellow, gray, green, or red. Sizes of the lesions vary; many coalesce to produce lesions up to 4 cm in diameter. Typical histomonic liver lesions are also diagnostic. Some have a radial spoke-like appearance.

Diagnosis of histomoniasis can be based on history, clinical signs, and typical lesions in a few freshly dead, or moribund birds. Although the organism dies soon after the bird dies, it can usually be demonstrated in birds killed at necropsy. The organism is found in large numbers at the edges of cecal lesions or in scrapings from the edge of liver lesions. Also the organism can be demonstrated in stained tissue sections of the liver lesions.

Supportive laboratory procedures should be conducted to differentiate the disease from other infections, e.g., coccidiosis, paratyphoid, aspergillosis, and trichomoniasis. The histomonad can be cultured but most diagnostic laboratories are not equipped for culturing; therefore, diagnosis is based on typical gross and microscopic lesions.

TREATMENT AND CONTROL:

FDA's withdrawal of legal-use clearance for Emtryl (dimetridazole) and Ipropan (ipronidazole), the two most effective drugs for treating histomoniasis, dealt a severe blow to poultry producers. Currently the only effective drug available for treatment of outbreaks is Flagyl (metronidozale). Flagyl is a drug developed for treatment of humans but is also effective against avian intestinal protozoan flagettes. Flagyl can be obtained from a veterinarian or by prescription at a pharmacy. The dosage for large peafowl-type birds is is 250 mg daily or 1.5 g/gal in the drinking water for 5 to 15 days. Other treatments include copper sulfate (1:2000) or acidified copper in the drinking water for 5 days. Nonmetallic fountains must be used with the copper compounds. Nitrofuran drugs are helpful if available, but these drugs have been pulled from the market.

Feed for chukar and other highly susceptible species should be medicated with Histostat, a feed-additive drug. Mills having a FDA mix-clearance on file to may legally add Histostat to its poultry feed.

Control of histomoniasis outbreaks requires a coordinated approach: medication of the outbreak flock by feed and/or water, eliminating the cecal worm (by deworming the flock) to avoid reinfection, by replacing litter, and disinfecting floors of indoor pens. If birds are on wire, administer the medication and wash floor with high-pressure detergent solution.

In early Spring, before vegetation emerges or new birds arrive, treat all outdoor pens with Benomyl [3 lb/acre] to kill earthworms, then till pens superficially (to a depth of only an inch or two). Benomyl may be used, at the approved rate, when birds are in the pens.

PREVENTION:

Good management and good sanitation are the best prevention for histomoniasis, especially with birds in pens with floors of concrete. Pens should receive thorough C& D before each new brood. After brooding, chukar partridges and other highly susceptible species should be grown on wire. Most chukar producers eventually build wire-floor pens in order to minimize histomoniasis and the birds' contact with droppings, cecal worm eggs, and earthworms. Other preventive measures include: controlling cecal worms, not mixing gamebirds with chickens or using pens frequented by chickens, cultivating soil to control earthworms in dirt pens, medicating feed with Histostat, performing rigorous C& D of pens after each flock, selecting outdoor pens with sandy, dry, loose soil, and putting feeders and fountains on wire-floor platforms.

LEUCOCYTOZOONOSIS

DEFINITION:

Leucocytozoonosis is a malaria-like disease of birds, affecting primarily birds on range. It is caused by an arthropod-borne protozoan that enters the blood stream, damaging blood cells and tissues. The disease is characterized by sudden onset, anemia, and enlargement of the spleen and liver. Acutely affected birds die.

The causative organism is a leucocytozoon species-protozoan blood parasite. At least 100 species have been identified; 10 or more of these are found in North America. Most species are host specific so cross-infection is not a threat. Recovered birds remain carriers.

Like the coccidia, leucocytozoon undergo several developmental stages. As with malaria protozoa, fertilization and sexual development of this parasite occurs in the body of the insect vector (black fly or biting midge).

Infected birds and the insect vectors serve as reservoirs of the disease over winter. Acute outbreaks have been reported in most species of domestic waterfowl and in wild turkeys. It seems that birds are intermediate hosts of the parasite. Birds of any age are susceptible, but the disease is more damaging in young birds. Ducks, geese, and turkeys on range are the bird species most often infected. Common species of the parasite are *Leucocytozoon simondi* (waterfowl), *L. neavel* (guinea fowl), *L. andrewsi* (chicken), and *L. smithi* (turkeys).

Infected gamebirds are usually seen with distorted erythrocytes, leucocytes, or with distorted RBC and WBC together. Birds appear to be the only hosts of most Leucocytozoons. In the United States, leucocytozoonosis occurs most frequently from the midwestern states eastward along the Atlantic coast, particularly in the southeastern states. There are few reports of the disease in other countries.

TRANSMISSION AND CLINICAL SIGNS:

Leucocytozoonosis is transmitted by black fly species (simulium species) and by biting midges (culicoides). Wild or domestic birds that survive the disease are carriers during the winter. During the warmer season, vector insects feed on carriers, taking in the leucocytozoons.

The protozoa undergo sporogeny (i.e., formation of sporozoites) in the host insect and pass to the host's salivary glands. The insect vectors are blood feeders and when they feed, the leucocytozoons are transmitted to the host bird. Surviving birds become carriers.

The insect vector remains infective for about 18 days. The disease does not spread bird-to-bird nor is it spread by egg transmission. Clinical signs will appear within a week of exposure and include sudden onset, severe anemia, fever, weakness, rapid labored breathing, loss of appetite, dullness, lameness, green diarrhea, and neurological malfunctioning. The course is often quick and infected birds either die or begin to recover within a few days.

High mortalities occur in acute outbreaks. Death is caused by blockage of vital vessels with large meronts (developmental parasites) or respiratory distress caused by blockage of lung capillaries, and anemia from blood loss. Chronically affected birds are unthrifty in growth and production.

LESIONS AND DIAGNOSIS:

Primary lesions are acute anemia and low white blood cell count, as well as hemorrhage and enlargement of the liver and spleen. In birds that survive for a few days, splenic enlargement may become the most pronounced lesion. The large white dots found in many organs are meronts. Severely anemic birds exhibit respiratory distress from the massive number of parasites that occupies the lung capillaries. Encephalitis lesions can be found in birds that showed incoordination before death. Gamonts (schizonts) are seen in thin blood smears along the edges and the tail of the smear. Shape of the gamonts will vary from round to long tapering extremities. There are no pigment granules in blood cells.

Also, microscopically, megaloschizonts are present in the brains of birds paralyzed or birds with loss of equilibrium. Smaller schizonts can be found in liver sections.

Presumptive diagnosis can be based on history of endemic leucocytozoonosis in the area, typical signs, lesions, and presence of protozoan blood parasites in blood smears. The clinical diagnosis is made by identifying the blood parasite in stained (Wright's and Griemsa) blood smears. Further confirmation is by histopathologic examination of blood smears. Wright's or Giemsa stain should be used to reveal developmental stages of the protozoan. Affected cells usually are enlarged in size and altered in shape by the gamete. Extensive damage to liver, spleen, brain, and lungs can be demonstrated.

TREATMENT AND CONTROL:

Effective treatment for stopping or controlling an outbreak does not exist, but a few drugs appear to minimize the severity of the disease.

Recommended prophylactic medications to control *L. caulleryi* in chickens include pyrimethamine [1 ppm] and sulfadimethoxine [10 ppm] in the feed; for control of *L. smithi* in turkeys, use clopidol (coyden [1.25 to 2.5 ppm] in the feed). Any one of these drugs is recommended for treating outbreaks of leucocytozoonosis in gamebirds and waterfowl.

Absolute control is not possible unless birds are grown indoors throughout their life, or where insect vectors are eliminated from the environment. The black fly will not enter buildings to feed; therefore, indoor confinement at least during the corresponding season for these particular insects will offer some control.

Both black fly and biting midge breed in rapidly flowing streams. The disease outbreaks occur following seasonal hatches of these insect vectors.

PREVENTION:

Minimize or eliminate exposure to insect vectors. If young birds are grown on range, get rid of adult birds before the insects hatch and before young birds are placed on the range. Without carrier birds, the black fly remains free of leucocytozoon, and therefore cannot transmit the disease.

If wild carrier birds are present, eradication of the disease is not possible. For birds kept in indoor confinement, install fly-tight screens on openings to keep out the biting midge (i.e., the vector for *L. caulleryi* in chickens). Black flies generally will not enter buildings to feed, thus keeping ducks, geese, turkeys, and other susceptible gamebird species confined indoors during the vector's breeding season should avoid exposure.

PLASMODIUM INFECTIONS

DEFINITION:

Plasmodium infections are acute protozoan parasitic infections (malaria) that affect the red blood cells of poultry. The infections are transmitted by mosquitoes and cause severe anemia, weakness, and death. Protozoans of the genus Plasmodium that infect red blood cells (RBC) of poultry are the cause of this disease. Plasmodium is closely related to the genera Haemoproteus and Leucocytozoon, but plasmodia replicate in circulating RBC — in contrast to the endothelial cells and leucocytes with the haemoprotei and the leucocytozoa, respectively. Plasmodia contain pigment.

Malaria outbreaks in North America are more often found in Anseriformes (ducks), Passeriformes (songbirds), and Columbiformes (pigeons). Plasmodium species tend to have a preferred host, but some cross-infection does occur. Approximately six species of plasmodium that prefer domestic fowl (chickens, turkeys, pheasants, and guinea fowl) have been identified. A number of passerine Plasmodium species, on occasion, have infected domestic fowl. *P. gallinaceum, P. juxtanucleare,* and P. *durea* appear to be the species most dangerous to chickens, turkeys, and ducks.

Avian malaria is prevalent in wild birds in the United States, but is of low economic importance in domestic poultry. All species of birds are susceptible, as are humans and probably other mammals. Malaria is more often acute in young poultry and more often chronic in adult birds. Avian species of plasmodia tend to be host-limited to host-specific. For example, *P. gallinaceum* infects domestic flocks; *P. cathemerium* infects aviary birds; and *P. relictum* infects wild birds and wood ducks.

About 65 Plasmodium species have been identified, and the pathogens infect more than 1000 species of birds. While the disease is diagnosed worldwide, the major outbreaks occur in Asia, Africa, and South America. Avian malaria is diagnosed throughout the world, primarily in the spring, summer, and fall in the colder climates. In temperate climates, where the insect vector can breed year-round, the disease becomes a year-round problem.

TRANSMISSION AND CLINICAL SIGNS:

Mosquitoes (Culex, Ades, and Anopheles species) infected with plasmodia spread the disease when they feed on the avian host. The life cycle of this pathogen requires two hosts, i.e., the bird and the mosquito. The bird is considered to be the intermediate host.

Asexual development and generation of immature sexual forms occurs in the red blood cells of birds. Fertilization and sexual maturity of this protozoan occur in the mosquito, the final host. Avian malarial infections have been induced experimentally by administering the protozoan parasite to experimental birds by mouth.

The mosquito bite is the natural route of transmission. The disease is characterized by sudden onset, severe anemia, marked weakness, labored breathing upon mild exertion, loss of appetite, brief illness, and in acute cases, death. A few birds within the flock may develop paralysis from capillary blockage in the brain. Canaries exhibit swelling in the region of the eyes. Mortality may reach 90 percent in acute outbreaks.

LESIONS AND DIAGNOSIS:

Malarial lesions are similar to those of toxoplasmosis. Since the disease involves blood cells, the most striking lesion is anemia. Gross lesions include subcutaneous hemorrhage and swelling of the spleen and liver. Microscopic examination shows infarction (blockage) of small vessels. Laboratory confirmation is based on the demonstration of the Plasmodium parasite in RBC of stained blood films or in smears from suspect birds.

Laboratory procedures such as the microhematocrit will measure the severity of anemia. Comprehensive blood studies should be made on several birds in a suspect flock. The disease, as seen in RBC in blood films stained with Romanowsky stain, exhibits a signet-ring effect. The Plasmodium-infected RBC consists of a thin ring of protoplasm with a nucleus at one side. The center of the parasite (comprising the bulk of the cell) is vacuolated and does not stain. The ring (i.e., the protoplasm) and the nucleus stain blue, thus presenting the ring-like appearance.

TREATMENT AND CONTROL:

Chemotherapy is used in treating affected individuals or flocks of pigeons, caged songbirds, and penguins. Successful treatment of flocks requires breaking the life cycle of the parasite by eliminating or controlling the mosquito. The highly pathogenic plasmodium species are found in Africa and Asia. Quarantine and import controls reduce the risk of importing infected fowl.

Effective treatments for certain bird species include: chloroquine [250 mg/4 oz drinking water, grape juice, or orange juice]. Grape or orange juice will cover the bitter taste of the drug; chloroquine [5 mg/kg body weight daily in fish] is preventative for penguins. Any of the antimalarial drugs, including pyrimethamine, quinine, clopidol (coyden), and sulfadimethoxine at the dosage prescribed for leucocytozoonosis [10 ppm in feed] are recommended.

PREVENTION:

Since malaria is transmitted by infected mosquitoes, mosquito control is the key to prevention. Some of the antiprotozoal agents give some relief to malaria-infected birds. Atabrin, Pyrimethamine, and clopidol have efficacy against malaria and leucocytozoon diseases. Check drug package label for dosage and use restrictions. But make mosquito control your first line of defense against plasmodium problems.

SARCOSPORIDIOSIS

DEFINITION:

Sarcosporidiosis is a parasitic disease, primarily of ducks, reptiles, and mammals. The disease is caused by protozoa of the genus Sarcocystis. The parasite localizes in the skeletal muscles and is characterized by cysts in the muscle. Synonym for Sarcosporidiosis is Sarco. *Sarcocystis rileyi* is the primary pathogen infecting ducks and other birds.

Birds are intermediate hosts for sarcocystis parasites. The opossum is the definitive host to one or more of the avian Sarcocystis. The pathogenicity of Sarcocystis species in birds is not known. Birds (except perhaps ducks) with apparently heavy infections of this parasite may be asymptomatic. Experimentally induced infections in ducks will produce signs of illness. Younger ducks, by virtue of their young age and lack of acquired resistance, are more susceptible than mature ducks.

One report on susceptibility lists susceptible birds of 19 genera, 20 species, and 13 families. Therefore, the host range is quite diverse. Although gallinaceous and passerine birds can be infected, they obviously are not the preferred host of the parasite.

Sarco is probably of greater economic importance in its effect on birds in the wild than on domestic fowl. Ducks appear to be the only class of poultry economically affected by this parasitic disease. Sarco occurs worldwide. Precise distribution is not known because much of the reporting is that of incidental findings on various types of birds when autopsied. Sarco infections have been reported in a number of birds significant to the Audubon Society.

TRANSMISSION AND CLINICAL SIGNS:

Sarco is thought to spread in the feces of carrier birds. Sarcosporidiosis is most prevalent in hosts (birds/others) that drink from shallow stagnant pools. Further transmission is from feed and water contaminated with sporocysts (i.e., the organism in its asexual stage).

There is no conclusive evidence that Sarco is spread by a vector. The stable fly has been implicated in spread to mammalian hosts, but not to birds. Even so, invertebrate hosts such as beetles, aquatic organisms, and even other forms of internal parasites (such as nematodes), are possible invertebrate hosts.

All avenues of transmission have not been identified, but it is known that the opossum and small rodents serve as definitive hosts. Clinical signs of Sarco are vague or lacking. Even in controlled experiments, the signs are often vague or nonspecific. The disease is often found in birds that appear normal. It has been reported that sarco-infected ducks fly low and slowly, implying loss of vigor. Signs and lesions in mammals are more conspicuous, and include unthriftiness, emaciation, skin irritation, lameness, incoordination, and death.

LESIONS AND DIAGNOSIS:

Gross lesions found at necropsy are multiple (often massive) and white, giving a speckled effect to the pectoral muscles, especially in ducks. Microscopic tissue changes have been described as fatty degeneration of the muscles, enlargement and occasional rupture of parasitized fibers, and inflammation of surrounding muscle tissue.

The marked pathological changes, i.e., glomerular and tubular nephritis noted in cattle, sheep, and swine have not been reported in birds. Sarco bodies are positioned lengthwise to the muscle fiber of the breast, thigh, neck, and/or esophagus. Lung hepatization and enlarged spleen are the major changes in the organs.

Diagnosis is confirmed by identifying the protozoan parasite in fixed and stained muscle tissue of an infected bird. Muscle tissues should be sectioned at 10-μ thickness and fixed, using standard procedures, in Bouin's fluid or other fixatives, and stained with hematoxylin-eosin. The parasite stains blue. Direct microscopic examination can be done on fresh, unstained muscle tissue by compressing finely minced tissue between glass plates, then examining under high magnification. Sarco bodies are elongate and will be seen within the muscle fiber.

TREATMENT AND CONTROL:

Potassium iodide, sulfadimethoxine, and amprollium all will show efficacy toward Sarcocystis. The histomonastat and antimalarial drugs may also be helpful. Arsenic is very toxic to waterfowl, so drugs containing arsenic (histomonastats and other) must be avoided. Initiate tight biosecurity measures to prevent pen entry by predator mammals (mink, raccoon, skunk, opossum, etc.); these animals are likely to contaminate feed, water, and the pens.

Follow generally recommended husbandry and management practices to assure healthy birds. Do not use medications that are knowingly toxic to bird species that might gain access to the medicated feed or water. Follow manufacturer's guidelines for drug withdrawal for slaughter or release of birds medicated.

PREVENTION:

Prevention requires sanitation, isolation of known infected areas, and control of predators, rodents, and insects. Since the life cycle of Sarcocystis is not completely known, control of predators and employment of proven management practices to prevent contamination of poultry feed and water is essential.

TRICHOMONIASIS

DEFINITION:

Trichomoniasis is a serious protozoal disease of gamebirds, pigeon, doves, fowl, and raptors. The disease occurs in two manifestations, i.e., in the upper and lower digestive tracts. The UPPER FORM is characterized by caseous lesions of the mouth, pharynx, esophagus, and crop. The LOWER FORM is characterized by muco-catarrhal enteritis and diarrhea. Common names for the upper form are canker, roup, and frounce. The causative agents are *Trichomonas gallinae* (UPPER) and *T. gallinarum* (LOWER) form. Both species have flagella and an undulating membrane used for locomotion. Most game, domestic, and caged birds are susceptible.

The disease is most serious in young birds. Pigeons, doves, and raptors are more susceptible to the UPPER FORM. The pigeon and dove transmit *T. gallinae* to their young in crop milk. Pigeon growers and falconers readily recognize *T. gallinae*. Gallinaceous birds are more susceptible to the LOWER FORM, *T. gallinarum*. The disease occurs wherever birds are grown throughout the world and is widespread in the United States, where it occurs mostly as sporadic outbreaks.

TRANSMISSION AND CLINICAL SIGNS:

Transmission is bird to bird or by contact with contaminated feed, water, or litter. Pigeons are the primary carriers. Pigeons contaminate water and feed with oral secretions and transmit the disease to their young by crop milk. Pigeons and other free-flying birds may spread trichomonas to gamebirds and domestic poultry who probably contract the disease by drinking from stagnant pools. Recovered birds remain carriers. Clinical signs of the UPPER FORM include drooling (greenish mouth fluids), depression, sunken empty crops, stretching neck motions with frequent swallowing, open-mouth breathing, and fetid mouth odor. The UPPER FORM, rarely seen in turkeys, is found primarily in gamefowl chickens, and occasionally in gamebirds. Clinical signs of the LOWER FORM of trichomoniasis are depression, unkempt appearance, watery yellow diarrhea, loss of weight, and death. These clinical signs are also suggestive of histomoniasis.

LESIONS AND DIAGNOSIS:

UPPER FORM: Lesions are confined to the mouth, pharynx, esophagus, and crop. Typically, there are yellow plaques or raised caseous masses that are large, conical, or pyramidal which may make closure of the mouth difficult. Most lesions are in the mouth and esophagus but lesions have been reported in the crop, stomach, lungs, and sinuses.

LOWER FORM: Lesions are primarily in the intestine, ceca, and liver. The condition may be confused with histomoniasis. In pheasant and chickens, there is a pronounced muco-catarrhal enteritis. Intestinal contents are a creamy yellow texture. In peafowl and turkeys, there is a caseous core, cecal distention, and necrosis. Liver lesions are raised, granular, and yellow in color. Diagnosis is based on typical gross lesions, history, clinical signs of behavior, odor, and posture. Microscopic demonstration and identification of the organism confirm the diagnosis. Diagnostic lesions of the UPPER FORM are the canker and presence of *Trichomonas gallinae* in the saliva. Diagnostic lesions of the LOWER FORM are enteritis, liver lesions, and *T. gallinarum* in the intestinal or cecal smears.

TREATMENT AND CONTROL:

Medication for the UPPER FORM and the LOWER FORM is the same, because *Trichomonas gallinae* and *T. gallinarum* are sensitive to the same drugs. Any protozoacide is usually effective. These drugs [Flagyl (metronidazole), copper sulfate solution (1:2000), and acidified copper] are those prescribed for histomoniasis.

The LOWER FORM may respond to nitrofuran drugs. Emtryl (Dimetridazole) or Ipropan (Ipronidazole) is recommended when available. Carnidazole, available in small-dose tablets, is approved and effective for pigeon and dove, BUT IS NOT RECOMMENDED FOR OTHER BIRDS.

Drugs and dosages listed for histomoniasis are recommended for either form of trichomonas, including pigeon and dove, if carnidazole is not available.

For control of trichomoniasis during outbreaks, rely on good sanitation, husbandry, and biosecurity measures. Use separate caretakers for adult and young birds. Sanitize footwear and hands upon leaving a bird pen. Keep dead and moribund birds removed and incinerated. Clean and sanitize waterers at least once daily. Do not save breeder replacements from infected flocks. C& D pens after each flock.

Employ recommended hatchery sanitation procedures even though trichomonas is not egg-passed. Administer and monitor medication judiciously. Examine dead birds to monitor effectiveness of medication.

PREVENTION:

Most of the general measures for disease control apply to prevention of trichomoniasis. Other measures include depopulation at regular intervals and C& D of premises. Eliminate sickly birds and suspect carrier birds.

Eliminate stagnant water pools in the pen and always provide clean fresh water. Do not add mature birds to an established flock. Do not permit contact among pigeon, dove, raptors, and poultry. Do not feed infected pigeons and doves to raptors. Periodically medicate flock with a protozoacide.

GROWER'S REFERENCE

ON

GAMEBIRD HEALTH

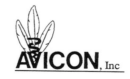

AVICON, Inc

INTERNAL PARASITES OF GAMEBIRDS

OVERVIEW

Helminth parasitism occurs naturally in all types of birds including song, terrestrial, and waterfowl, as well as all species of domestic and gamebirds. During a necropsy, many species of worm parasites are found in the digestive tract as well as in other organs. Numerous species of parasites are cause of concern for the damage that they inflict upon their hosts There are two major classes of internal worm parasites. The roundworms or nematodes are nemathelminthes. The flatworms or cestodes and trematodes are platyhelminthes. To establish control methods, accurate diagnosis (i.e., accurate identification of the species) is essential.

Knowledge of the life cycle of the parasite is also essential. Nematodes have either a direct or an indirect life cycle. Treatment for species with direct life cycles is focused on the natural host. By contrast, parasites with indirect life cycles (cestodes, trematodes, and some nematodes) require effective two-part control procedures: (i) interruption of the intermediate host and (ii) anthelmintic treatment of the bird to expel the parasite.

In terms of numbers and damage, nematodes are the most important group of helminth parasites. Nematodes are called roundworms because the worms are spindle-shaped, nonsegmented organisms with a smooth cuticle or body covering. Some may have transverse grooves. With few exceptions, nematodes are sexually distinctive. The male is distinguished by the presence of two chitinous spicules at the caudal end of its body. By contrast, cestodes (tapeworms) are not sexually distinctive since they are hermaphrodites.

Nematodes pass through four developmental stages in the process of becoming adults. The eggs pass in the droppings of the infected birds, embryonate in the environment, hatch in the proventriculus of hosts, and undergo larval growth to maturity. Serious tissue damage is done by the larvae. Many penetrate and migrate through tissues before maturing and returning to the digestive tract of the bird. The tissue trauma increases the susceptibility for localized bacterial infections from multiple tissue-puncture wounds. Tissue damage also permits the loss of blood and tissue fluids, perhaps leading to anemia. Most nematodes feed on blood.

Platyhelminth flat worms, especially tapeworms, inflict damage by living in the host bird's digestive tract and competing for digested food nutrients. The worms have no digestive tract, and therefore must rely on their host to digest the food that is then absorbed by the worm. Tapeworms attach to the mucosal surface of the wall and extend down the intestine. In competition with the host, the worms absorb nutrients flowing through the intestine.

Birds and animals with heavy tapeworm infections maintain hearty appetites but lose weight because the tapeworms get the food.

ANTHELMINTICS

A variety of commercially available anthelmintics are effective and safe to use in eliminating nematodes (common round worms, cecal worms, gapeworms, *Capillaria*, etc.) and tapeworms from gamebirds. FDA regulations, however, limit the use of certain compounds when used in birds. Drugs currently approved as well as drugs for which clearance may soon be granted are listed here. Remember to always follow FDA regulations and carefully read the product label for the manufacturers' instructions on use of all products.

ROUTE	ANTHELMINTIC	BRAND NAME
Feed	Hygromycin **B**	Hygromix
Feed	Levamisole^	Tramisol
Feed	Coumaphos	Meldane-**2**
Feed	Fenbendazole^	Safeguard
Feed	Piperazine	Several brands
Feed	Phenothiazine	Several Brands
Feed	Butynorate^^	Tinostat
Feed	Triple dewormers	Wormal
Feed	Triple dewormers	Worm-a-floc
Feed	Thiabendazole	TBZ
Water	Piperazine	Several brands
Water	Levamisole^	Tramisol
Wet Mash	All of the above	

^Clearance for poultry pending

^^ For turkeys only

ASCARIDIA

Ascaridia, the common round worm, is the most prevalent of the worm parasites of gamebirds. It causes heavy economical losses each year. Roundworms do the most damage to the bird during their migratory or tissue phase of development..

Larval ascarids migrate within the mucosa (lining) of the intestine. The migration causes a hemorrhagic type of enteritis with a severe adverse effect on the bird. The parasitized bird is unable to digest or assimilate feed efficiently; thus, growth is retarded. Producers need to pay special attention to the control of the ascarid in every young flock.

Ascarids are large, thick, yellow white worms with heads having three distinct lips. The male measures 50 to 60 mm and the female 60 to 116 mm in length.

It has been known since 1788 that the ascarid parasite is species specific, with little or no cross-infection from one class of poultry to another. Most classes of domestic birds have their own species of ascarid worm that likewise is host-specific. *Ascardia galli* is the chicken ascarid; *A. dissimilis* is the turkey ascarid; *A. numidae* is the ascarid for the guinea fowl; and *A. columbae* is the pigeon ascarid. One exception is *A. galli*, the chicken ascarid, which can cross-infect, at a low rate, turkeys, doves, ducks, and geese.

LIFE CYCLE:

The life cycle of the chicken ascarid is simple, direct, and may require only 35 days. The adult female worm, while in the host bird, lays eggs that pass out with the feces and embryonate (i.e., reach larval stage) in the litter. Viable worm eggs in the litter germinate (i.e., become infective) within 5 days. The optimum germination temperature is 90 to 93°F. Chickens ingest the infective eggs while pecking in the litter. The ascarid eggs then hatch in the stomach of the birds and the larvae pass into and live freely in the intestine. On day 9, the larvae penetrate the mucosa. The tissue (i.e., migratory) phase extends from the 9th to the 17th day, when the ascarid re-enters the lumen of the intestine. By the 34th day, the worms are mature and begin laying eggs. Mature worms remain in the lumen of the intestine until death. The life cycles of other ascarid species are similar, but have not been studied to the same detail as *A. galli*.

Young poultry are the most susceptible to worm damage. At 2 or 3 months of age, the bird develops resistance (cell-mediated immunity) to the ascarid. The mature bird can tolerate a few adult ascarids without damage. For example, ten worms per hen are considered not harmful, but more than 75 worms per hen will cause damage.

PATHOLOGY:

One of the primary effects of ascaridia infection is weight and growth depression in the host bird. Heavily parasitized birds are anemic, unthrifty, weak, and more susceptible to infectious diseases. Heavily parasitized birds, because of their weakened condition, are unable to generate an optimum immune response to vaccinations. In severe infections, blockage of the intestine may occur. Ascarids are intestinal worms but they have been found in other parts of the body such as the abdominal cavity and the oviduct. Ascarid worms occasionally migrate up the reproductive tract where they become trapped within the egg.

CONTROL:

As the ascarid worm is a litter-borne parasite, it is not usually a problem in birds reared on wire. However, flies can transport the worm eggs from manure pits to birds in cages; thus *A. galli* can become a problem in the caged-poultry house. Control is best accomplished by combining medication with management. Several anthelmintics (wormers) eliminate this worm from the intestines of the birds, but drugs alone do not give total control. For example, young birds reared on new litter in sanitized buildings will be protected with a single medication at 35 to 40 days of age.

Birds reared on reused or built-up litter should be medicated twice, at 4 and again at 6 weeks. The medication should be timed to eliminate the worms before they reach maturity at 35 days, thus interrupting the life cycle of the parasite. In floor-raised replacement birds, the flock should be first wormed at 5 weeks of age and again at 30-day intervals until 21 weeks of age — a total of at least four wormings.

Piperazine, the most common anthelmintic used for ascarids, is safe at ten times the recommended dosage. Piperazine expels the ascarids from the lumen of the intestine and they soon die.

Adult worms and nonembryonated eggs are not infective when eaten. Reinfection is established only if the bird ingests infective worm eggs. Use only FDA approved wormers as recommended. Vitamin A fortification of the feed for 5 to 7 days will speed healing of the intestinal mucosa damage caused by ascarid migration. Most wormers are administered in the feed for a single day of treatment. Give Piperazine in the drinking water [35 to 50 mg/lb bird's body weight] for one day.

CAPILLARIA

Seven species of Capillaria worms infect gamebirds, pigeons, ducks, geese, and domestic poultry. *Capillaria annulata* and *C. contorta* are parasites of the crop and esophagus. *C. obsignata, C. bursata, C. caudinflata,* and *C. columbae* are parasites of the small intestine. *C. retusa (anatis)* infects the ceca. Ova are oval-shaped and operculated (i.e., having an operculum) on both ends. Worm sizes are 8 to 17 mm for males and 15 to 60 mm for females. Worms appear to be threaded into the mucosa of the infected organ.

Birds heavily infected with *Capillaria* become culls. A typical history of layer flocks infected with *Capillaria* will have an excessive number of cull birds as well as a general decrease in production. Pigeons are unthrifty, become weak fliers, and in general perform poorly. Birds retain appetites but do not respond to antibiotic therapy. The comb regresses as the bird becomes anemic and emaciated. Eggs from infected hens have pale, mottled yolks due to low vitamin **A** content.

When infected birds are necropsied, *Capillaria* worms may be found. Presence of *Capillaria* ova in scrapings of the digestive tract or feces confirm a presumptive diagnosis. If the crop is infected, it will have thickened walls and be void of feed but will contain an excessive amount of mucus substance. If the infection is intestinal, the duodenum and/or cecum will be acutely inflamed.

LIFE CYCLE:

Life cycles of *Capillaria* species are described as "direct"or "indirect". The earthworm serves as the intermediate host (IH) for capillaria, heterakis, and syngamus. *Capillaria* nematode eggs pass in the droppings of the bird. Incubation (i.e., embryonation) requires 24 to 30 days. The egg becomes infective only in the embryonated form.

Transmission is specific for each capillaria species. For example, *C. obsignata* and *C. bursata* have direct transmission. Birds become infected only when they eat feed, drink water, or ingest scratchings from litter or soil contaminated with embryonated eggs of these two species.

Gamebirds, ducks, turkeys, and chickens can become infected with the severely harmful *C. annulata* or *C. contorta* in either manner; that is by ingesting embryonated eggs directly, or by eating an earthworm that has ingested embryonated eggs of these two nematodes.

Earthworms that eat embryonated eggs become infective. Completion of the life cycles of *C. caudinflata* and *C. columbae* requires the involvement of the intermediate host. Only embryonated eggs ingested by earthworms are harmful. This is the explanation for the occasional diagnosis of these two capillaria species.

PATHOLOGY:

Young birds heavily parasitized with *Capillaria* tend to huddle in isolated areas. Infected birds may be emaciated, have diarrhea, and hemorrhagic enteritis before death. With intestinal capillariasis, the gut wall thickens and the mucosa becomes hemorrhagic with bloody catarrhal exudates. The intestinal damage interferes with digestion, feed utilization, and performance.

Even though birds show the clinical signs of anemia (pale tissues, shrunken comb, lethargy), there is no significant change or loss of red or white blood cells. Blood from pigeons infected with *Capillaria* shows decreased total protein and serum albumin. Thus, the anemia is the result of decreased protein and albumin in the blood.

Reductions in plasma carotene and vitamin A levels occur in the livers of birds with heavy *Capillaria* infections. Eggs from infected hens have mottled yolks because of the vitamin A deficiency. With crop capillariasis, the tissue pathology is similar to that of intestinal capillariasis; however lesions are confined to the crop, esophagus, and lower pharynx. Quail and other gamebirds are more susceptible to crop than to intestinal capillariasis.

CONTROL:

Coumaphos is the only medication that is approved and consistently effective against *Capillaria* species. WARNING: COUMAPHOS TENDS TO BE TOXIC TO PHEASANTS. Hygromycin B at 12 g/ton of feed for 12 weeks provides some action against *Capillaria*. Thiabendazole (TBZ) is effective against *Capillaria* species and is FDA-approved for gapeworms in pheasants. Tramisol (levamisole), soluble in water, is an effective anthelmintic against *Capillaria* and other poultry nematodes, but levamisole requires an 8-day withdrawal period to allow time for residues in the eggs to abate.

Experimentally, Fenbendazole is effective with doses of 54 g/ton of feed for 5 to 7 days. Supplemental vitamin A (6,000 to 2,000,000 IU/bird/day) has been used with some benefit. Hematinic compounds (i.e., stimulators of RBC formation) are helpful. Other less-specific medicants are Polystat (as recommended for coccidiosis) and Thiabendazole (454 g/ton of feed for 14 days). BUT. . .Thiabendazole and Polystat may not be used on meat birds within 30 days of slaughter.

KNOW AND HEED ALL WARNINGS for any wormer that is used. Pyrantel tartrates, Thiabendazole, Fenbendazole, and Mebendazole are anthelmintics that will become of value against Capillaria species when approved by the FDA.

Good management is an absolute requirement for successful control of *Capillaria*. The infection cycle must be broken. This is accomplished by strict sanitation and flock isolation. Recommended procedure is to depopulate, clean up, disinfect, steam the floor (steam at 141°F kills eggs of *Capillaria* species). Then restart the production cycle. Always use good management procedures with proper sanitation and isolation to avoid re-infections. Applications of insecticide or compounds lethal to earthworms and soil nematodes will disrupt the life cycles of *Capillaria* worms. Quail and chukar partridge should be grown on wire to avoid infection with Capillaria or contact with other possible infectious diseases.

CHEILOSPIRURA

Cheilospirura are gizzard worms that commonly infect quail, grouse, partridge, pheasant, chickens, turkeys, and guinea fowl. It is the most frequently encountered of the gizzard worms. There are other genera of nematodes, however, that produce gizzard worms in these bird species, as well as in ducks, geese, pigeon, and doves. The other nematode genera are: Amidostomum (four species), Echinura (two species), and *Cvrnea neeli, Cyrnea eurycerea, Epomidiostomum uncinatum,* and *Streptocara crassicauda*. The genera Amidostomum has a direct life cycle (LC) while the intermediate hosts of other genera range from grasshopper, beetle, water flea, amphipod, or is unknown. Cheilospirura, the most prevalent gizzard worm uses the grasshoppers and beetles as intermediate hosts (IH). Genus identification becomes important in diagnosis because effective treatment and control require the elimination of the IH. Only Cheilospirura will be specifically addressed. All other genera will have similar life cycles. Treatment and control measures would be the same.

The natural hosts of C. *spinosa* include grouse, partridge, pheasant, quail, and wild turkey. The worms are found in the gizzard beneath the corneous lining. The worms have four spiny cord-like organs occurring as pairs that originate between the lips and extend to the upper third of the esophagus. These structures, easily seen under low power magnification, are important in the worm's identification. The Worm lengths are 14 to 20 mm for the male and 34 to 40 mm for the female. The male has spicules of unequal size on its tail or caudal end. The vulva of the female is anterior to the middle of the body. Size of the worm egg is 27 to 42 μm (millimicron).

LIFE CYCLE:

Cheilospirura is thought to have originated in the grouse, then spread to infect quail. Now it is known to infect grouse, turkey, guinea, partridge, and pheasant, as well as quail. Gizzard worms have been parasites primarily of free-ranging birds in the wild and not a problem in birds grown in confinement.

Birds on the range have easier access to the infected intermediate host(s). The IH for *Cheilospirura* is the grasshopper and beetle; it is in these insects that worm development progresses to third-stage (i.e., infective stage) larva. Larvae eaten before reaching the third-stage of development are not infective. In quail, the fourth-stage larvae were found beneath the gizzard lining 14 days after the bird has ingested the infective larvae. Maturation and LC completion were seen by 32 days postinfection. Worm eggs were found in the feces, which is in itself a sign of completion of the life cycle.

PATHOLOGY:

Today, quail appear to be the gamebird species most often infected with *Cheilospirura*. The probable explanation is that high numbers of quail are produced annually. The southern climate is conducive to quail and to the nematode. Light infections cause minimal problems in quail, even though tortuous worm migration trails are found beneath the gizzard lining in the gizzard muscle. Heavy infections, by contrast, cause the gizzard lining and muscle to become hemorrhagic and necrotic. Chronic sign of infection is proliferative tissue changes in the gizzard muscle. The diagnosis of gizzard worms in any gamebird operation should be followed by prompt control measures. Gizzard worm infections impact on the health and hardiness of the birds. Birds will be less thrifty and poorer performers in growth and flight.

CONTROL:

Primary control measures require that birds be monitored for the presence of gizzard worms. A necropsy examination to check for worms can be done whenever a bird dies from any cause. During routine necropsy, open the gizzard, examine the contents, then remove the lining. Gizzard worms will be beneath the lining and burrowed into the muscle. If worms are present, several unthrifty birds should be submitted to a diagnostic laboratory for gizzard worm diagnosis and identification.

In the meantime, treat all flocks in outdoor dirt pens with an anthelmintic. Phenothiazine, Fenbendazole, TBZ, and Tramisol wormers are helpful. A grasshopper- and beetle-control (i.e., IH- control) program should be started by mowing weeds around the outside of the pens. Then apply of Sevin or Malathion to a swath 50 to 100 feet in width around the pen perimeter. In quail operations where IH control is not effective, the birds should be grown on wire and kept off the ground in infected pens. Growers should always check with entomologists at the State University for a control program for the IH species.

DISPHARYNX

All forms of dispharynx worms recovered from galliform, columbi-form, and passeriforme birds appear to be identical, with nonspecific host; therefore, all are classified as *Dispharynx nasuta*. *D. nasuta* is the only species of this genus. Natural or definitive hosts are quail, par-tridge, grouse, pheasant, pigeon, passerine birds, chickens, turkeys, and guinea fowl. Dispharynx worms parasitize the upper digestive tract, they are found in the wall of the proventriculus, sometimes in the esophagus, but rarely in the intestine. Morphologically, disphar-ynx worms have wavy folds on the head area that contain four cord-like cardon structures that appear like the esophagus of the nematode. The cardons extend to the end of the fold and turn back to mid-point of the fold. When not in tissue, the nematode maintains a coiled or spiral position. The worms measure 7 to 8 mm in length for the male and 9 to 10 mm in length for the female. The eggs are embryonated when laid.

LIFE CYCLE:

The genus *Dispharynx* has an indirect life cycle (LC). Pill bugs and sow bugs of the *Isopod* genus serve as the intermediate hosts (IH) for the *Dispharynyx*. The embryonated eggs hatch within 4 days after being eaten by an IH. Larvae escape and can be found among the tissues of the body cavity. Larvae complete development in 26 days. Larvae are then infective, and will mature and complete the LC when eaten by a susceptible bird host. Infective larvae are also called third-stage lar-vae. When eaten by the definitive host, the female nematode develops to sexual maturity, deposits eggs in 27 days, and thus completes the LC in 57 or 58 days.

PATHOLOGY:

Dispharynx nematodes are found with their heads buried deep into the mucosa. Ulcers and local inflammation are present at the attach-ment site. The nematode has a predilection for the proventriculus and the wall becomes markedly thickened and the bird emaciated. The parasites are almost completely concealed beneath the proliferating tissue. *D. nasuta* is the chief cause of "grouse disease" in the northeast-ern USA. Heavy infections cause death in pigeons. Wild pigeons, trapped at Balboa Zoological Park, San Diego, California, were heav-ily infected with *D. nasuta*. Quail more than other captive gamebird species tend to be seriously infected with the nematode. Because of the wide range of hosts *D. nasuta* tends to remain endemic in areas where, once established, cause annual health problems in gamebirds and poultry.

CONTROL:

In control, the goal becomes to interrupt the life cycle of the worm by destroying the intermediate hosts. Precise knowledge of the drug sensitivity of *Dispharynx* is limited. However, control of the intermediate host (pill bug and sow bug) is probably of greater importance. Birds can then be treated with an approved anthelmitic (wormer) that should kill and expel the parasite. Thiabendazole and related wormers are considered to be the most effective against *Dispharynx* in birds.

It is essential to emphasize biosecurity and good husbandry that, in pens known to be infected, includes thorough C&D between flocks The soil should be treated with a safe, FDA-approved pesticide that will control the IH before susceptible birds are released into the area.

GONGYLONEMA

Gongylonema ingluvicola is the only parasite of this genus that infects avian species. The more prevalent bird hosts are quail, pheasant, partridge, chickens, and turkeys. *Gongylonema* worms attach and burrow into the mucosa of the esophagus, crop, and proventriculus. The crop is the preferred site. Morphologically, adult worms have shield-like markings in a longitudinal arrangement on the end with the head. The markings are scattered on the head but are numerous and in longitudinal rows. Male worms are 17 to 20 mm long. The females are 32 to 55 mm in length, and wider than the male. The male is distinguishable by the cervical papillae on the head and two narrow bursal membranes on the tail. Also, the male genital spicules are uneven in length. Barbed points are located at the end of the tail. The vulva of the female is positioned 2.5 to 3.5 mm from the tip of the tail.

LIFE CYCLE:

Beetles and cockroaches serve as intermediate hosts for the *Gongylonema*, thus the life cycle is indirect. In an experiment, chickens ate larvae collected from beetles and only a single male worm was recovered. In another experiment, larvae were collected from mountain quail. Subsequently, cockroaches were infected with these third-stage larvae and fed to chickens. When the chickens were necropsied 12 weeks later, they were free of worms. Chickens appear to be more resistant than quail to *Gongylonema*. *Gongylonema* nematodes are rarely found today. Modern husbandry and sanitation practices have effectively controlled this potentially serious parasite.

PATHOLOGY:

The primary damage associated with *Gongylonema* nematodes is the trauma to local tissues in the mucosa of the crop, esophagus, and proventriculus. The burrow trails appear as white convoluted tracks in the mucosa and crop. The lesions may be confused with those of capillaria worms unless they are examined under low power microscopy. The *Gongylonema* worms must be differentiated from other nematodes (*Capillaria, Dispharynx, Tetrameres, Echinura, Cvrnea*, and *Physaloptera*) that infect the crop, esophagus, and proventriculus.

CONTROL:

Control of the *Gongylonema* is direct and simple. Treat infected birds with a benzimidazole carbamate (TBZ, Safeguard, Albendazole) wormer. Simultaneously, upgrade the environmental hygiene. Use pesticides to control beetles and cockroaches. When the outbreak is confined indoors, replace litter and treat the floors with Sevin (carbamate) or some other pesticide approved for poultry premises. If infection persists, contact a poultry pathologist to prescribe treatment for the birds and an entomologist to make recommendations for control of the beetles and cockroaches.

HETERAKIS

Heterakis gallinarum is commonly known as the cecal worm since the worm localizes in the ceca. Geographically, the parasite is found in all major areas of chicken, turkey, gamebird, and waterfowl production. Cecal worms cause nonspecific clinical signs of infection such as general unthriftiness, ruffled feathers, depressed appetite, and reduced growth rate. The worm is small, slender, and white. The head end is bent upward and the mouth is surrounded by three small lips. Two membranes extend almost the full length of the body. Adult worms measure 2 to 8 mm long.

The worm is important because of its role in the spread and perpetuation of histomoniasis. There is only one Heterakis species but it infects a variety of bird species. The worm eggs pass in the feces, germinate in the litter, then are ingested by the birds. In one report, egg numbers per female worm were greatest in ring-neck pheasants, followed by guinea fowl, turkeys, and chickens.

LIFE CYCLE:

The life cycle of histomoniasis begins when the organism *Histomonas meleagridis*, a protozoan, is picked up by the cecal worm in the intestine of an infected bird. The cecal worm then produces *H. meleagridis*-infected eggs that pass in the bird's droppings and germinate into infective larva. Earthworms feed on infected heterakis eggs. The eggs then hatch in the digestive tract of the earthworm and become encysted in the wall of the earthworm. Infective cecal worm eggs or infected earthworms may be ingested by gamebirds, turkeys, and other birds as they feed. The *Histomonas* organism is once again in the intestine of a bird, and the heterakis-histomoniasis cycle is repeated.

PATHOLOGY:

The ceca of experimentally infected birds show inflammation and thickening of the walls. In very heavy infections, nodules may form in the mucosa and submucosa. Actual bird losses have not been attributed, per se, to heterakis. The chief economic importance of *Heterakis* lies in its role as a carrier of *Histomonas meleagridis*. Histomoniasis may be produced in susceptible birds by dosing them with embryonated *Heterakis* eggs taken from infected birds.

CONTROL:

Control should be coordinated for both heterakis and histomonas. Medicate flock with known effective wormers such as phenothiazine, hygromycin B, or Meldane-2 (coumaphos) to eliminate cecal worms. These drugs are about equal in effectiveness. Follow label instruction on the drug and use only as approved by FDA. New anthelmintics known to be active against Heterakis should be considered as FDA approves them and they become commercially available. Anthelmintics currently under FDA clearance trials include Fenbendazole, Thiabendazole, and Mebendazole. All poultry anthelmintics have some use-restrictions required by law and must not be used indiscriminately. After medication, move the flock to clean, noninfected pens. For histomoniasis control, see under "Protozoan Diseases."

ORNITHOSTRONGYLUS

Ornithostrongylus quadriradiatus is an internal parasite primarily of pigeons and doves in the United States. The nematode is found in the lumen of the small intestine. The worms are delicate, slender, and (when freshly collected) red from the ingestion of blood. The cuticle on the area of the head inflates to form vesicular enlargement. In size, the males are 9 to 12 mm and the females 18 to 24 mm in length.

The male has a bilobed bursa that bifurcates near the tip to form two short tips with a blunted process on each side of the base. The genital spicules are curved with each terminating in the shape of a three-tine fork. The vulva of the female is near the end of the tail and is accompanied by two muscular ova ejectors. The tail tapers to a narrow blunt end with a short spine. The eggs are embryonated when deposited.

LIFE CYCLE:

Ornithostrongylus are blood-eating nematodes that inhabit the small intestine of pigeons and doves. The eggs are oval, thin-shelled, and pass in the feces of the bird. Worm eggs hatch in 19 to 25 hours when environmental conditions are favorable. The larvae molt twice within the first 3 to 4 days to reach the third (i.e., infective) stage.

The infective larvae are ingested, along with contaminated feed, water, or litter by the host. Within a week, the worms are mature and begin laying eggs. A life cycle may be as short as 12 to 14 days.

Ornithostrongylus nematodes are capable of creating serious outbreaks in pigeon or dove lofts. The life cycle is direct; that is, the eggs embryonate and are infective within the environment of the host. This creates the opportunity for multiple generations of worms with potential for heavier total infections to the birds.

PATHOLOGY:

Ornithostrongylus causes a severe catarrhal hemorrhagic enteritis, with loss of blood, in the heavily parasitized birds. Total bird loss is high in severe outbreaks. Since the life cycle of *Ornithostrongylus* is short and direct, the potential for massive outbreaks is great.

Spread occurs by direct contact with infected birds, droppings, or contaminated feed, water, and litter. Spread is likely during "homing" contests or bird shows. Heavily infected birds are weak, and lethargic. They remain squatting on the ground or floor and, if disturbed, tend to tip forward on the breast and head.

The birds refuse food and become anorexic. Food eaten is often regurgitated with bile-stained (greenish) fluid. At the same time, infected birds develop a greenish diarrhea, lose weight, and die. Labored breathing precedes death.

Intestines of dead birds are mucoid, greenish, and have hemorrhagic enteritis with clumps of sloughed mucosal epithelium. Histopathologically, intestinal tissues of dead birds are necrotic. The intestinal wall in the infected area is void of mucosa. Worms may be demonstrated in the tissue section.

CONTROL:

Absolute control requires depopulation, thorough C&D of facilities, and rest for the facility before repopulating. A treatment-control program requires treating the birds with a Benzimidazole (TBZ, Safeguard) wormer, C&D of premises, and monitoring the flock for residual infections. Repeat the treatment-control cycle each month as long as infection is evident.

While treatment-control procedures are going on, do not mix resident and feral birds. Do not participate in flight or homing trials or bird shows until the infection is eradicated. Notify other local pigeon and dove fanciers that *Ornithostrongylus* is present and suggest that their birds be examined by a laboratory.

OXYSPIRURA

Oxyspirura mansoni is an eye worm. Bird hosts for this parasite include quail, grouse, pigeon, peafowl, guinea fowl, ducks, turkeys, and chickens. Wild birds are usually the source for this parasite. The worm is found in the eye beneath the nictitating membrane (third eyelid), conjunctival sacs, and nasolacrimal ducts.

Both ends of the worm are tapered and cuticle is smooth, without membranous appendages. The circular mouth is surrounded by a five-lobed chitinous ring with two lateral and four submedian papillae. The worms have two pairs of dorsal and one pair of ventral teeth. The male is 8 to 60 mm in length, has a ventrally curved tail without alae, but has four pairs of preanal and two pairs of postanal papillae. The genital spicules are of unequal length. The female is 12 to 20 mm long. The eggs are embryonated when laid. There have been over 70 species of *Oxyspirura* described, most of which were from wild birds.

LIFE CYCLE:

Oxyspirura has an indirect life cycle, with the cockroach serving as the intermediate host. Eggs from mature females are deposited into the eye of the host bird. Eggs wash down the tear ducts, are swallowed, and pass in the feces. The cockroach, an omnivorous feeder, ingests the eggs. The eggs hatch, mature, and migrate to the abdominal cavity of the cockroach. Within 50 days, the larvae become encysted in the tissues of the insect host. When the insect host is eaten by a susceptible bird, the nematode larvae are freed in the crop, migrate up the esophagus to the mouth, then by way of the nasolacrimal duct reach the eye. A variety of wild birds, especially the black bird, feral pigeon, shrike, and blue jay have been experimentally infected with the worm, but the infection occurs naturally in sparrows, doves, coturnix quail, and pheasant.

PATHOLOGY:

Oxyspirura eyeworms cause severe conjunctivitis, opthalmitis, and protrusion of the third eyelid. Eye exudates cause the eyelids to stick together. The eye tissues become inflamed and swollen, and protrude. The bird appears to be uneasy and continuously scratches the eye to dislodge the worm. This physical reaction may actually remove the worm, as worms are rarely found in the eyeball — even those with severe signs. If left untreated, the bird develops severe opthalmia that destroys the eye. Another eye worm species, *O. petrowi,* is found in upland gamebirds; *O. petrowi* is also known to infect a wide variety of wild birds. The lesions are identical to the lesions caused by *O. mansoni*. All pathology is confined to the eye. Secondary bacterial infections increases the problem in that they lead to blindness in the birds.

CONTROL:

Control is achieved by establishing a control program for the cockroach. This requires thorough C&D of premises, a cockroach-control program, and treatment of the flock with a systemic anthelmintic. Recommended anthelmintics are Tramisol, Ivermectin, or TBZ. Repeat C&D and flock treatment on a monthly basis and continue the cockroach-control program throughout the insect season. Tighten biosecurity. Keep birds segregated by age and species. Minimize cross traffic. These programs should be in effect year round. Obtain a laboratory confirmation of the worm species. Consult with an avian pathologist for flock medication recommendations and an entomologist for a cockroach-control program.

SYNGAMUS

Syngamus trachea, gapeworm, is a nematode that infects the trachea of poultry and other birds. Gapeworms, also referred to as "redworms," (due to their color after a blood meal) and "forked worms" (male and female are attached in permanent copulation). Gapeworm is a red, round, worm that causes the disease known as the "the gapes." "Gapes" is descriptive of the open-mouth breathing of birds infected with gapeworms. Heavily infected birds usually emit a grunting sound because of difficulty in breathing. Many birds infected with gapeworms die from suffocation. Gapeworms grow rapidly and soon block the trachea, so the condition is particularly harmful to young birds. Gapeworm infections affect chickens, turkeys, guinea fowl, pheasants, chukar partridge, and probably other birds. *Cyathostoma bronchialis* is the causal organism of gapes in ducks and geese.

LIFE CYCLE:

Life cycle of the gapeworm can be either direct or indirect. Earthworms are the primary intermediate host, as is the case with the cecal and the capillaria worm. The parasite is ingested when birds eat embryonated eggs of the syngamus worm or feed on earthworms that have eaten gapeworm larvae. The mature female gapeworm lays eggs while in the lumen of the trachea of the bird. The eggs are coughed up, swallowed by the bird, and subsequently passed out in the droppings.

The actual migration of *Syngamus* larvae from the intestine to the lungs was not understood until 1965. Then researchers reported that larvae enter the blood stream from the duodenum and are carried to the lung. Larvae have been found in liver and lung tissues, as well. Apparently the larvae molt in the lung, then enter the bronchi, and migrate up to the trachea. Mature gapeworms have been found in the trachea as early as 4 days after experimental infection and firmly attached to the trachea within 11 days.

Gapeworm eggs embryonate within 8 to 14 days on the ground or in litter. Embroyanated eggs become infective when eaten by birds, earthworms, or other intermediate hosts. In the intermediate host, gapeworm larvae hatch and become encysted (blister-encased) in the muscle tissues. Earthworms remain infective to birds for up to 4 1/2 years, and in snails and slugs for up to 1 year. When the intermediate host is eaten by a bird, encysted larvae hatch in the intestine, migrate to lungs, and ultimately into the trachea to repeat the life cycle. Development to mature worms occurs as early as 4 days after ingestion of *Syngamus* larvae.

PATHOLOGY:

Gapeworms present a serious problem in pen-raised pheasants and in turkeys grown on range. *S. trachea* is the worm that infects the gallinaceous birds. *Cyathostoma bronchialis* is the gapeworm of ducks and geese. Young birds are most seriously affected. The worms grow so rapidly that they obstruct the lumen of the trachea. Experimentally inoculated Guinea fowl, pigeons, and ducks did not exhibit characteristic signs of infection.

Clinical signs include weakness, open-mouth breathing with "grunting" sounds, and emaciation. Birds sit with their heads drawn back and eyes closed. Severely infected birds do not eat, and will convulsively shake their heads to dislodge the worms. The tracheal mucosa is inflamed and the irritation causes coughing. Nodules found in the trachea of pheasants and turkeys are points of permanent attachments of *Syngamus* nematodes. *Syngamus* females remain in permanent copulation attachment with the male, although she may detach herself from the tracheal wall in search of food. Blood consumption by the worms is minimal, so the main damage to birds is through mucosal injury, air blockage of the trachea, and suffocation.

CONTROL:

Gapeworms are primarily a problem in young birds reared on infected soils in range pens. The condition is seldom diagnosed in chickens and only occasionally in turkeys confined in buildings. With pen-raised pheasants, gapeworms are a very serious problem. Some control or reduction in infection density (worms per bird) is achieved by using specific pens only on alternate years and/or by restricting a pen to a single brood each year. Broods reared successively in pens already infected contribute rapidly to buildup of gapeworm population.

Tilling pens with dirt floors at the end of the growing season helps to destroy residual infection. Soil-sterilization compounds will destroy earthworms, snails, and slugs, but the cost is usually prohibitive. Chemicals designed for controlling soil nematodes in orchards and on vegetable farms are available and are cost effective.

Gapeworms develop resistance or tolerance to a drug after about 2 years of repeated usage. Therefore, choice of drug and frequency of use should be tailored to individual pens. In general, birds in pens known to be infected should be dewormed at 15- to 30-day intervals. Drug dosage and frequency of treatment must comply with FDA-approved clearances. Treat farm-wide for the specific condition in the pen.

Thiabendazole [454 g/ton] in feed for 14 days is FDA-approved for treatment of pheasants.

Levamisole, a soluble drug not yet FDA-approved, is commonly used for gapeworm treatment in poultry and gamebirds. It is administered [1 g/gal] in the drinking water for one day. Repeat after 7 to 14 days.

Fenbendazole, a new drug for broilers, turkeys, and pheasants, is currently in process for FDA approval. Fenbendazole [54 g/ton] is effective when administered in feed for 5 days.

Treat pens with Benomyl [3 lb/acre] to control earthworms before spring tilling or replacing birds.

TETRAMERES

Tetrameres nematodes are stomach worms that parasitize most game-bird species, domestic fowl, and waterfowl. *Tetrameres* species have indirect life cycles in which the grasshopper and cockroach are the intermediate hosts. *Tetrameres crami* infects only ducks and the amphipod is the intermediate host. Other species of the genus are *T. americana, T. fissispina, T. pattersoni* (quail), and *Microtetrameres helix* (infects only pigeons). Followinng discussion pertains to *T. americana,* the most common species diagnosed. The range of hosts for *T. americana* is quail, grouse, ducks, turkeys, and pigeons. The parasite was named by Cram in 1926.

Tetrameres, primarily a parasite of free-ranging birds or birds confined to outdoor pens, is the common stomach worm found in quail in the southern regions. In current-day production of domestic poultry, *Tetrameres* is not an economic entity; therefore, gamebirds, by nature of being grown outdoors become the target host for this nematode. Quail appear to have a greater susceptibility to *Tetrameres* than do the other gamebird species.

The adult worm assumes a rounded shape. The worm burrows into the stomach wall. When the bird is necropsied, worms can be observed through the wall of the organ. On the surface of the stomach, the parasite appears as a small blood blister with the body of the worm buried in the tissues.

Morphologically, the mouth of *Tetrameres* has three lips and a buccal or mouth cavity. The male is 5 to 5.5 mm long, slender, with two double rows of spines running the full length of the body. The globular-shaped female is blood red in color, and 3.5 to 4.5 mm long and 3 mm wide. The uteri and ovaries are long with coiled configuration. The ova, embryonated when laid, measure 42 by 50 μm (millimicron). It is the female worm that is seen on the exterior surface of the stomach wall, with an appearance resembling a hematoma.

LIFE CYCLE:

Tetrameres have indirect life cycles. Grasshoppers and cockroaches are intermediate hosts. The nematode male is small and slender and is found on the surface of the stomach mucosa. Usually the male enters the gastric glands only to mate with the female. In some birds, however, the male is found with the female in the stomach gland. In this instance, both nematodes are permanent residents within the gland.

The eggs are embryonated when laid. Eggs fed to grasshoppers produced infective larvae in 6 weeks. The worm larvae were found in the body cavity of the insect. When the infected insect is eaten by the bird, the larvae escape and undergo molt to the fourth-stage nematode. Females enter the gastric glands, mate, and produce embryonated eggs by 45 days postinfection.

The life cycle, in general, is 3 months or longer. The parasite is perpetuated season to season in infected birds. Each spring, new susceptible intermediate-host insects become infected as they ingest the embryonated eggs from the feces of infected birds.

PATHOLOGY:

Infected birds become emaciated and anemic as a result of the heavy parasite loads. In chickens, the walls of the proventriculus may be so thickened that the lumen is almost obliterated or closed. *T. americana* produced only mild infections in quail. However, *T. pattersoni*, the quail species, produced lesions and damage equal to that of *T. americana* in chickens In quail, the worms were so numerous that little or no healthy stomach wall remained. *T. americana* has been reported in feral and domestic pigeons. Heavy infections produce diarrhea, emaciation, and death. *T. fissispina* infects waterfowl and wild birds, but rarely infects domestic poultry. With any severe infection, reactions occur with degeneration of glandular tissue, edema, and leukocyte infiltration. The results are emaciation due to starvation, followed by a secondary bacterial infection. Pathology from *Tetrameres* nematodes is confined to the proventriculus.

CONTROL:

Tetrameres is a soil- and litter-borne disease caused by the parasite. The insect intermediate hosts become infected from ingesting worm eggs in the bird pens. New avian hosts become infected as they feed on infected grasshoppers and cockroaches. Control requires treating the birds to kill and expel the worms. This is followed with C& D of the pens, feeders, and other equipment to help to avoid re-infection of the intermediate hosts. Grasshoppers and cockroaches feed on the bird droppings as well as the bird feed.

Tetrameres worms are sensitive to the benzimidazole wormers (TBZ, Fenbendazole). On a monthly basis, repeat the treatment of the flock and pens. Segregate birds by age and species. Bring new hatches into pens only after thorough C& D.

Tetrameres must be differentiated from other stomach worms, i.e., *Dispharynx, Cyrnea, Echinura, Physaloptera,* and *Gongylonema.*

TRICHOSTRONGYLUS

Trichostrongylus tenuis is an intestinal and cecal nematode of quail, pigeon, guinea fowl, chickens, turkey, ducks, and geese. The nematode was described by Mehlis in 1846 and was classified as a *Trichostrongylidae*. The worms are small and slender; the upper body is tapered. The mouth is surrounded by three small lips. The cuticle is smooth and void of the striations found on nematodes of a similar size. The male ranges from 5.5 to 9 mm in length. The male has a ventral cuticular inflation in front of the bursa that contains lateral lobes which have a fan-like appearance. The female is 6.5 to 11 mm in length. The vulva is at the posterior end of the body and has crenelated edges. The eggs are smooth with a thin shell.

LIFE CYCLE:

T. tenuis is the only avian species of this nematode with a direct life cycle (LC). The life cycle is completed within the natural host. Ova are passed in the feces of the bird, then germinate and hatch in the environment. The larvae live in the environment as free organisms, molt twice to become third-stage (i.e., infective) larvae. The germination and hatching process requires 2 weeks under favorable conditions. Once germinated, infection begins as larvae are eaten by the bird. Once eaten, the larvae migrate to the cecum where they molt twice to reach maturity. The approximate time to maturity is 14 to 21 days. After maturation, the worms mate and the female commences egg production. Total life cycle under optimum conditions is 4 to 6 weeks.

PATHOLOGY:

T. tenuis was associated with the disease that decimated the red grouse in Scotland. A fatal dose can be as low as 500 infective larvae. The ceca becomes dilated and blood vessels become congested. The cecal mucosa becomes edematous, thickened, and inflamed with greatly thickened ridges. Heavily parasitized birds become anemic and lose weight. *T. tenuis* is fatal to young goslings. Heavy mortality is seasonal, in that it occurs primarily to the young birds in the fall. However, in pens that were not sanitized at the beginning of the year, mortality can be high in young birds in the spring. The chronic form occurs throughout the year.

If *Trichostrongylus* has ever been diagnosed on the farm, the parasite-control program should include provisions for its control. Obvious means of spread include transfer of infective eggs or larvae on unsanitized boots, clothing, and equipment, or introduction of infected birds (e.g., purchased breeders). Presence of *Trichostrongylus* should be confirmed by laboratory diagnosis, so as to differentiate from other nematode parasites that infect the lower intestine and ceca, especially worm genera of *Heterakis, Capillaria, Aulonocephalus,* and *Strongyloides.* Outbreaks cause serious bird losses and surviving birds are stunted and unthrifty

CONTROL:

Control of *Trichostrongylus* must be a part of a total worm-control program for infected farms. The direct life cycle of this parasite requires a greater emphasis on biosecurity, sanitation, and husbandry. Do not mix birds of different ages. Monitor the health of birds in each age group. Get a laboratory confirmation and strictly adhere to the prescribed treatment and control measures. Obviously, initial emphasis is on sanitation and clean-up to break the re-infection cycle. Regularly medicate the flock to prevent fatal infection levels. This nematode is sensitive to benzimidazole (TBZ, Fenbendazole) wormers. TBZ is the drug of choice as it is effective and FDA-approved for use in gamebirds.

Other good husbandry practices can enhance recovery and minimize stress to the birds. Provide clean, fresh feed and water, maintain temperature at optimum for brooding birds, cultivate outdoor pens for better sun exposure, and sterilize the soil. Flocks in known infected pens should be treated monthly throughout the growing season. Breeders should be treated before the next breeding season.

TABLES — 213

LISTINGS OF INTERNAL PARASITES AFFECTING OR POTENTIALLY AFFECTING GAMEBIRD HEALTH

- NEMATODES -

NOTE: The nematodes tables are adapted with the permission of Michael D. Ruff (author), and The Iowa State University Press.

- TAPEWORMS -

NOTE: Tapeworm listing developed by W. Malcolm Reid.

NEMATODES REPORTED FROM CHICKENS AND GAMEBIRDS IN THE USA

NEMATODE	LOCATION	INTERMEDIATE HOST	OTHER DEFINITIVE HOSTS
Baylisascaris procyonis	Brain (accidental parasite in chicken, turkey, partridge, quail)	Racoon	
Oxyspirura mansoni	Eye	Cockroach	Turkey, duck, grouse, guinea fowl, peafowl, pigeon, quail
Syngamus trachea	Trachea	None	Turkey, goose, guinea fowl, pheasant peafowl, quail
Capillaria contorta	Mouth, esophagus, crop	None or earthworm	Turkey, duck, guinea fowl, partridge, pheasant, quail
Capillaria annulata	Esophagus, crop	Earthworm	Turkey, goose, grouse, guinea fowl, partridge, pheasant, quail
Gongylonema ingluvicola	Crop, esophagus, proventriculus	Beetle, cockroach	Turkey, partridge, pheasant, quail,
Dispharynx nasuta	Proventriculus	Sowbug	Turkey, grouse guinea fowl, partridge, pheasant, pigeon, quail

(CONTINUES)

NEMATODE	LOCATION	INTERMEDIATE HOST	OTHER DEFINITIVE HOSTS
Tetrameres americana	Proventriculus	Grasshopper, cockroach	Turkey, duck, grouse, pigeon, quail
Tetrameres fissispina	Proventriculus	None	Turkey, duck, goose, guinea fowl, pigeon, quail
Cheilospirura hamulosa	Gizzard	Grasshopper, beetle	Turkey, grouse, guinea
Ascaridia galli	Small intestine	None	Turkey, duck, goose, quail
Capillaria anatis	Small intestine, cecum, cloaca	None	Turkey, duck, goose, partridge, pheasant
Capillaria bursata	Small intestine	Earthworm	Turkey, goose, pheasant
Capillaria caudinflata	Small intestine	Earthworm	Turkey, duck, goose, grouse, guinea fowl, partridge, pheasant, pigeon, quail
Capillaria obsignata	Small intestine, cecum	None	Turkey, goose, guinea fowl, pigeon, quail
Heterakis gallinarum	Cecum	None	Turkey, duck, goose, grouse, guinea fowl, partridge, pheasant, quail

(CONTINUES)

NEMATODE	LOCATION	INTERMEDIATE HOST	OTHER DEFINITIVE HOSTS
Subulura brumpti	Cecum	Earwig, grasshopper, beetle	Turkey, dove, duck, grouse, guinea fowl, partridge, pheasant, quail
Subulura strongylina	Cecum	Beetle, cockroach, grasshopper	Guinea fowl, quail
Strongyloides avium	Cecum	None	Turkey, goose, grouse, quail
Tricho-strongylus tenuis	Cecum	None	Turkey, duck, goose, guinea pigeon, quail

NEMATODES REPORTED FROM POULTRY OR COMMERCIALLY RAISED GAME BIRDS OTHER THAN CHICKENS

NEMATODE	LOCATION	INTERMEDIATE HOST	OTHER DEFINITIVE HOSTS
Cyathostoma bronchialis	Trachea	None or earthworm	Turkey, duck, goose, (chicken)
Cyrnea colini	Proventriculus	Cockroach	Turkey grouse, prairie chicken, quail, (chicken)
Tetrameres crami	Proventriculus	Amphipod	Duck
Micro-tetrameres helix	Proventriculus	Grasshopper	Pigeon
Amidosto-mum anseris	Gizzard	None	Duck, goose, pigeon
Amidosto-mum skrjabini	Gizzard	None	Duck, pigeon, (chicken)
Ascaridia columbae	Small intestine	None	Pigeon, dove
Ascaridia dissimilis	Small intestine	None	Turkey
Ascaridia numidae	Small intestine	None	Guinea fowl
Ornith-ostrongylus quadri-radiatus	Small intestine	None	Pigeon, dove
Heterakis dispar	Cecum	None,	Duck, goose

(CONTINUES)

NEMATODE	LOCATION	INTERMEDIATE HOST	OTHER DEFINITIVE HOSTS
Heterakis. isolonche	Cecum	None	Duck, grouse, pheasant, prairie chicken, quail
Capillana columbae	Large intestine	None	Pigeon, dove

NEMATODES REPORTED, FROM WILD BIRDS IN THE USA, THAT POSE A POTENTIAL PROBLEM FOR POULTRY AND COMMERCIALLY RAISED GAME BIRDS

NEMATODE	LOCATION	INTERMEDIATE HOST	DEFINITIVE HOSTS
Oxyspirura petrowi	Eye pheasant, prairie chicken	Unknown	Grouse, quail,
Singhfilarla hayesi	Subcutaneous	Unknown	Turkey, quail
Splendidofilaria calitorniensis	Heart	Unknown	Quail
Splendidofilaria pectoralis	Subcutaneous	Unknown	Grouse
Chandlerella chitwoodae	Connective	Unknown tissues	Grouse
Aproctella stoddardi	Body cavity	Unknown quail	Turkey, dove,
Cardiotilaria niles	Body cavity	Mosquito	Chicken
Echinura uncinata	Esophagus, gizzard, proventriculus, small intestine	Water flea	Duck, goose
Echinura parva	Proventriculus, gizzard	Unknown	Duck, goose
Tetrameres pattersoni	Proventriculus	Grasshopper, cockroack	Quail
Tetrameres ryjikovi	Proventriculus	Unknown	Duck
Cvrnea neeli	Proventriculus, gizzard	Unknown	Turkey

(CONTINUES)

NEMATODE	LOCATION	INTERMEDIATE HOST	DEFINITIVE HOSTS
Cyrnea pileata	Proventriculus	Unknown	Quail
Physaloptera acuticauda	Proventriculus	Unknown	Chicken, pheasant
Amidostomum acutum	Gizzard	None	Duck
Amidostomum raillieti	Gizzard	None	Duck, dove
Cheilospirura spinosa	Gizzard	Grasshopper	Grouse, partridge, pheasant, quail, turkey
Cyrnea eurycerea	Gizzard	Unknown	Pheasant, quail, turkey
Epomidiostomum uncinatum	Gizzard	None	Chicken, duck, goose, pigeon
Streptocara crassicauda	Gizzard	Amphipod	Chicken, duck
Ascaridia bonasae	Small intestine	None	Grouse
Ascaridia compar	Small intestine	None	Grouse, partridge pheasant, quail
Porrocaecum ensicaudatum	Small intestine	Earthworm	Chicken, duck
Capillaria phasuanina	Small intestine, cecum	Unknown	Partridge, pheasant, guinea fowl

(CONTINUES)

NEMATODE	LOCATION	INTERMEDIATE HOST	DEFINITIVE HOSTS
Capillaria tridens	Small intestine	Unknown	Turkey
Aulonocephalus lindquisti	Cecum, large intestine	Unknown	Quail
Aulonocephalus pennula	Cecum	Unknown	Turkey
Aulonocephalus quaricensis	Cecum	Unknown	Quail

POULTRY TAPEWORMS AND TAPEWORM
INTERMEDIATE HOSTS IN THE UNITED STATES

CHICKENS AND GAMEBIRDS (also infects quail, guinea, pheasants, and occasionally turkeys and peafowl):

TAPEWORM	PATHOGENICITY	LOCATION	INTERMEDIATE HOST
Amoebotaenia cuneata	mild	upper intestine	earthworm
Choanotaenia infundibulum	moderate	upper intestine	housefly, beetle
Davainea proglottina	severe	duodenum	slug, snail
Hymenolepis carioca	unknown	jejunum	stable fly, dung
Hymenolepis cantaniana	mild or harmless	jejunum	beetle
Raillietina cesticillus	mild or harmless	upper intestine	beetle
Raillietina tetragona	moderate severe	lower intestine	ant
Raillietina echinobothrida	moderate to severe	lower intestine	ant

TURKEYS (infects guinea fowl):

TAPEWORM	PATHOGENICITY	LOCATION	INTERMEDIATE HOST
Davainea meleagridis	unknown	duodenum	unknown
Drepanidotaenia watsoni	unknown		unknown
Imparmargo baileyi	unknown		unknown

(CONTINUES)

TAPEWORM	PATHOGENICITY	LOCATION	INTERMEDIATE HOST
Raillietina ransomi	unknown	middle	unknown
Raillietina williamsi	unknown	middle	unknown
Metroliasthes lucida	unknown	middle	grasshopper

DUCKS AND GEESE:

TAPEWORM	PATHOGENICITY	LOCATION	INTERMEDIATE HOST
Diorchis nyrocae	unknown	intestine	crustacean
Fimbriaria	unknown	intestine	crustacean
Fasciolaris fasciolaris	unknown	intestine	crustacean
Hymenolepis anatina	severe	intestine	crustacean
Hymenolepis compressa	unknown	intestine	unknown
Hymenolepis collaris	unknown	intestine	crustacean
Hymenolepis coronula	unknown	intestine	crustacean, snail
Hymenolepis lanceolata	severe	intestine	crustacean
Hymenolepis megalops	unknown	intestine	unknown
Hymenolepis parvula	unknown	intestine	leech

TAPEWORMS

Tapeworms (cestodes) are white or yellowish ribbon-like segmented flat worms. One of the smallest is about one-sixth inch long. *Raillietina* species may be as long as 12 inches when mature and have only a few segments. Tapeworms grow by forming new segments (called proglottids) just behind the scolex (head). The tapeworm attaches itself to the wall of the intestine with the scolex. As it grows, segments on its caudal (i.e., tail) end mature and break off, then leaving the intestine with the droppings. The excreted segments are filled with "eggs"—actually first-stage cestode larvae. Insects and other arthropods eat the excreted segments and become intermediate hosts for the parasite. At least eight species of tapeworm infect chickens and gamebirds, six or more species infect turkeys, and nine or more infect ducks and geese (see listing, p 222).

LIFE CYCLE:

The life cycle of the tapeworm is indirect — i.e., the worm lives part of its life in an intermediate host (IH), such as a snail, slug, beetle, ant, grasshopper, earthworm, house fly, or other organism. Many tapeworm species are quite discriminatory about intermediate hosts. For example, the IH of the *Raillietina cesticillus* tapeworm of chickens and gamebirds is limited to three or four species of the grain and ground beetles — other species will not do. Grain beetles live in poultry litter, eating spilled feed. Because of this, *R. cesticillus* is the most prevalent tapeworm species found in broilers and other confined chickens. Many of these same tapeworms are able to infect other avian species (pheasant, guinea, quail, and turkey).

Poultry become infected with tapeworms by eating IHs (insects, snails, etc.) that carry immature tapeworms in their bodies. Tapeworm development can progress only to a certain level within the IH. Completion of the life cycle is dependent upon ingestion of the larval tapeworm by its natural bird host.

PATHOLOGY:

Tapeworms do not produce extensive lesions or damage to the intestines. Tapeworms are intestinal parasites, harmful because they are nutritional competitors. A cestode does not digest its own food. Instead, it anchors itself to the inner wall of the bird's intestine, letting its segmented body dangle in the flow of digested material, absorbing nutrients before they can be utilized by the host. The clinical signs of tapeworm infection include general unthriftiness, dry and unkempt feathers, hearty appetite, and loss of weight. Tapeworm segments are found in the droppings.

Diagnosis of tapeworm infection and identification of the species is best done by crushing mature tapeworm segments on a microscope slide, using a coverslip. Examination under magnification will reveal characteristics of the "egg capsule," unique in each tapeworm species. Species identification is important in order to identify its intermediate host — insect or arthropod.

CONTROL:

Control of tapeworms requires a dual approach—i) control of the IH to prevent reinfection and ii) treatment of infected birds to rid them of tapeworms. Since effective control is dependent upon elimination of the IH, the tapeworm species must be identified in order to determine the IH. Once the IH is known, entomologists can recommend an effective pesticide and a method of control.

To eliminate tapeworms from the poultry flock, medicate with Tinostat (butynorate) or any of the triple worming compounds (see "Anthelmintics," p 187). All are effective against tapeworms, but butynorate is more effective because it is specific against tapeworms. An effective tapeworm anthelmintic (wormer) must destroy the worm's scolex — not just knock off the tail segments. If the scolex remains unharmed, new segments form and the bird is soon as parasitized as before treatment.

GROWER'S REFERENCE

ON

GAMEBIRD HEALTH

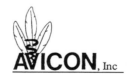

AVICON, Inc

EXTERNAL PARASITES OF GAMEBIRDS

OVERVIEW

External parasites of birds are arthropods that live on or in the skin and feathers. The insects breed and develop in the manure, dead carcasses, and moist organic materials — each an indication of poor sanitation. The external parasite problem has changed with the evolution of the gamebird and poultry industries.

Pests that were once common in small commercial and noncommercial flocks are less common today. Pests that spread bird to bird by body contact are more serious however, as bird density in the rearing and growing facilities has significantly increased. Control of external parasites requires the best possible management in integrated production operations. For example, the Northern fowl mite can survive for long periods away from its host. It can be transported on egg flats, crates, or clothing. Mites remain a major problem.

The house fly, a manure breeder, as well as a pesky nuisance can be a mechanical spreader of worm parasites. The fly carries worm eggs from the manure pit back to the birds in cages or adjacent pens.

Certain ectoparasites (lice) feed on dead skin cells and feather debris. Such parasites spend their entire life cycle on the host. Other pests, e.g., red mites and ticks, are nocturnal blood feeders that attack the birds at night. After feeding, these parasites move to daytime hiding places in cracks and crevices of nests, roosts, and walls. Some of the blood-feeding parasites harbor and spread infectious disease organisms.

Ectoparasites (i.e., external parasites) belong to different classification groupings. All belong to the animal phylum *Arthropoda* and are characterized by hard segmented bodies, jointed paired appendages, and chitinous exoskeletons. Lice, flies, bugs, fleas, and mosquitoes belong to the *Class Insecta*. Insects have three body parts — the head, thorax with three pairs of attached legs, and abdomen. Some adult insects have wings. Insects pupate, i.e., undergo metamorphosis from worm-like larvae to become adult insect parasites. Mites are members of the *Class Arachnida* characterized by the fused body with four pairs of legs attached to the abdomen. They are minute creatures related to the spider family. The female lays eggs that hatch as nymphs. Nymphs resemble the adult parasite but have three instead of four pairs of legs. Nymphs undergo a series of molts to become adults, then reproduce to repeat the life cycle.

Ticks are blood-sucking acarid parasites of the suborder *Ixodides*. Ticks are larger than their relatives, the mites. There are two families of ticks, the *Argasidae* or soft tick, and the *Ixodidae*, or hard tick. Life cycle stages of ticks are the same as those of for mites, with stages of eggs, nymphs, moltings, and adults. *Argas persicus*, the fowl tick, is a soft tick.

PESTICIDES[1] FOR CONTROL
OF EXTERNAL PARASITES

To protect users and consumers, all pesticides are regulated by state and federal laws Always read the labels carefully; follow instructions. Pesticides are toxic substances. Proper handling is essential. Store them in closed, clearly labeled original containers, out of the reach of children and animals. Keep pesticides in locked storage facilities.

Do not store pesticides in the same room with feed additives or medications. Do not allow pesticides to come in contact with the skin. Do not use ona windy day. Do not smoke, especially when handling pesticides. Do not inhale dusts, sprays, or vapors. Always wash hands and face after the use of pesticides.

APPLICATION	CHEMICAL[2]	EXAMPLES[3]
Premise sprays	permethrin	Permectrin II, Expar Ectiban, Permaban, Atroban
	carbaryl	Sevin
	tetrachlovinphos	Rabon
Residual premise sprays	diethyl diphosphorothioate	Malathion
	carbaryl	Sevin
	tetrachlovinphos	Rabon
	tetrachlovinphos & dichiovos	Rabon-Vapona
Animal sprays	permethrin	Atroban, Expar, Ectiban, Permaban, Permectrin II
	carbaryl	Sevin (several formulations)
	tetrachlorvinphos	Rabon
	coumaphos	Co-Ral
	tetrachlorvinphos & dichlorvos	Rabon-Vapona
		(CONTINUED)

[1] Adapted from 1993-94 Pesticide Recommendations for Poultry in Pennsylvania

[2] Pesticides approved by FDA and EPA

[3] Listing of trade names is for example only, and is not to be considered an endorsement

PESTICIDES[1] (CONTINUED)

APPLICATION	CHEMICAL[2]	EXAMPLES[3]
Animal dusts	permethrin	Permectrin
	permethrin	Permectrin strips
	carbaryl	Sevin
	diethyl diphosphoro-thioate	Malathion dust
Litter dusts	carbaryl	Sevin
	tetrachlorvinphos	Rabon

[1] Adapted from 1993-94 Pesticide Recommendations for Poultry in Pennsylvania

[2] Pesticides approved by FDA and EPA

[3] Listing of trade names is for example only, and is not to be considered an endorsement

BED BUGS

In fiction, the bedbug, *Cimex lectularius*, was a traditional pest of cow-town boarding houses, annoying gunman and lawman alike. In fact, bedbugs attack poultry and mammals, as well as humans. Poultry houses and pigeon lofts may become heavily invaded. *Cimex lectularius* hide, breed, and lay their eggs in nests, behind nest boxes, under loose boards, and in cracks about the walls, roosts, and roofs of poultry houses. Bedbugs are seldom found on fowl in the day time because, as blood feeders, they come out of hiding at night to feed on the sleeping birds. Setting hens are especially vulnerable, and may leave their nests if the bugs are numerous. Small black spots, excreta of the bed bug, are visible on eggs or in cracks. Heavily infested birds may become anemic.

Mature bed bugs are wingless, reddish-brown, and about 1/4 inch in length. The oval body is quite flat until engorged with blood. The female will deposit from 70 to 200 eggs in daytime hiding spots. The eggs hatch into nymphs in 6 to 17 days. The nymphal stage feeds for 1 to 2 months before maturing.

Bed bugs prefer warm environments and thus are more prevalent in temperate and subtropical climates. In colder climates, bedbugs are seldom a winter-time problem except in heated buildings. They survive for long periods without feeding. Infestations in poultry flocks usually are not observed until the poultry-house workers themselves develop inflamed welts and itching.

Treatment should be directed toward the daytime hiding places of the bed bug. Spraying the birds will also be helpful. If the infestation is heavy, total control requires treating the house and all contents at clean-out time. Success requires use of a residual chemical in combinaion with a fumigant to flush the bugs from their hiding places. Always use FDA-approved pesticides and fumigants.

BLACK FLIES

Several species of black flies attack poultry. The small, gnat-like, humpbacked flies swarm about the heads of fowls, piercing the skin and sucking blood. Along with painful biting, these pests can carry Leucocytozoon parasites that cause a malaria-like disease among turkeys and ducks.

Development of the black fly requires swiftly flowing water. Mature flies lay eggs on the surfaces of rocks, sticks, or vegetation in the stream. The eggs hatch into grayish-black, legless maggots within 2 to 12 days. The maggots (larvae) attach to obstructions in the flowing stream where water will surge over them. They transform into the pupal stage in 1 to 6 weeks. The pupal stage hatches in about 2 days to 3 weeks. The adults emerge, float to the water surface, and quickly take wing to begin feeding.

Simuliids are most troublesome in the northern part of the temperate zone and subarctic regions. Reports in the United States date back to the last century when buffalo gnats were noted to swarm on poultry. This forced chickens, turkeys, gamebirds, and waterfowl to leave their nests. Some black fly species travel several miles to seek a blood meal. Disease transmission by gnats to poultry was demonstrated in Nebraska where buffalo flies spread Leucocytozoon to turkeys.

Control is difficult because of the breeding habits of the insect. Insecticides may be harmful to fish. Area-wide control programs, using biological control agents such as Bacillus bacterial culture, have been developed Biological control requires weekly treatment of breeding areas within the large geographical region. Control of black fly control at its breeding sites may not be attainable. However, gamebird producers can establish some control in the brooding and growing areas by using repellent sprays to discourage entrance of the black fly into the facility. Blood protozoan parasites may be carried over winter in adult birds. The new generation of insect vectors then becomes infected when feeding on resident birds. The gamebird grower can prevent annual outbreaks of Leucocytozoonosis by disposing of adult gamebirds before onset of black fly breeding. Current gamebird hatches are not infected; therefore, even though the black fly or buffalo gnat feeds on birds it remains uninfected and as such is unable to spread or perpetuate the disease.

FLEAS

Fleas, order Siphonaptera, are parasites in the adult stage, but as larvae are free-living organisms. Adults vary in size from 1.5 to 5 mm. Fleas have a tough chitinous covering and are compressed laterally (thin shape). The mouth parts are designed to puncture skin and to siphon. Fleas have short antennae and long legs adapted to jumping. They are found worldwide, but are more abundant in the warmer climates. The life cycle varies, depending upon temperature, humidity, and host availability. Fleas can survive long periods without feeding. Birds returning to infested former nesting or roosting areas become infested with fleas. Six species of fleas have been found on birds but only three species of significant economic importance have been reported in North America.

STICKTIGHT FLEA: The sticktight flea, *Echidnophaga gallinacea*, is prevalent in the southern United States, though occasionally it is found in the northern states. Adult fleas attach in clusters up to a 100 or more to the skin of the head and embed their mouth parts. Once embedded, the fleas are very difficult to dislodge. The adult flea remains attached for days to weeks. The female forcibly ejects her eggs into the environment.

The natural bird hosts of fleas are pheasant, quail, chickens, turkeys, pigeons, blackbirds, bluejays, hawks, owls, and sparrows. Fleas also feed on mammals as well as most domestic and wild animals. The sticktight fleas do not transmit infectious diseases to gamebirds and poultry. Experimentally, the sticktight flea did transmit the typhus agent of humans to guinea pigs and other laboratory rodents.

EUROPEAN CHICKEN FLEA: The European chicken flea, *Ceratophyllus gallinae*, has been reported in the northeastern United States. Its hosts are gamebirds, poultry, pigeons, and songbirds, as well as humans and most rodent animals. The flea stays on birds long enough to feed. Immature forms are often found in the nesting areas of birds.

WESTERN CHICKEN FLEA: The western chicken flea, *Ceratophyllus niger*, is found primarily on the west coast of the United States and in Alberta, Canada. It attacks most bird species, mammals, humans, confined gamebirds, poultry, as well as feral birds, gulls, and cormorants. The appearance and life cycle are the same as for the European chicken flea.

OTHER FLEAS: The cat flea, *Ctenocephalides felis*, invades poultry houses where cats are used to control rodents. The fleas breed in the poultry house and then move onto the birds. The squirrel flea, *Orchopeas howardii*, occasionally invades the poultry house. Likewise, the human flea, *Pulex irritans*, will attack birds when hungry.

LIFE CYCLE:

Similar to insects, fleas have four life-cycle stages — egg, larvae, pupae, and adult. Adult female fleas deposit several white spherical eggs each day, these roll from the host into the nest or litter to incubate. The eggs hatch in one to two weeks as worm-like larvae that feed on the feces of fleas and organic matter in the litter, feather sheaths, and skin scales of birds. Fully grown larvae spin a cocoon to pupate, then emerge as young fleas. Newly emerged fleas seek a host, suck blood, and become sexually mature within a few days. Immature fleas may live for weeks or months without food. Adult fleas can live up to a year without food if hosts are unavailable. The life cycle varies, depending upon the environmental circumstances as well as the availability of hosts. Similar life cycles are characteristic of most species of fleas.

PATHOLOGY:

It is as blood feeders that fleas are most damaging — especially to skin and feathers. Heavy infestations in nesting and young birds will cause the birds to become anemic, perhaps fatally. Secondary infections result from the skin damaged by feeding fleas. Fleas, at least as far as is known, do not spread infectious agents as do mosquitoes, black flies, and biting midges. Besides anemia, feather damage, and skin irritation, fleas stress the birds by creating general discomfort. Most flea species attack the host to feed but the sticktight flea remains attached for days or weeks, thereby causing more health problems for the infested birds.

CONTROL:

Flea control requires the elimination of the parasite from the environment. The most important measures are removal of the litter followed by a thorough spraying of the house with a poultry-approved pesticide to kill the immature fleas. In most cases, the building should be cleaned and disinfected, then followed with the pesticide application. Without C& D, remaining flea eggs will hatch and reestablish the flea population. Monitor routinely for fleas.

The approved pesticides listed (p 231) are effective against fleas. In Scotland, pyrethroid permethrin was effective against the European chicken flea when it was sprayed in nest boxes and litter at 0.125 to 0.25% concentration.

HOUSE FLY

Musca domestica, the common house fly, is a serious pest, health, and sanitation problem for gamebird and poultry operations. House flies are non-biting flies that breed in animal droppings, manure piles, spilled feeds, and other decaying organic matter. Adults feed on manure or animal secretions through sponging mouth parts that project downward from their heads. The life cycle is as short as 7 days under ideal conditions. Each female can produce 120 to 150 eggs, laid in six or more batches, at 3- to 4-day intervals.

Fly control in and around poultry operations is usually a serious problem. Even though flies cause no direct damage to birds, they are efficient carriers of disease and filth, and thus become a public nuisance. House flies are also considered to be intermediate hosts for certain poultry tapeworms and indirectly perpetuate ascarids in caged birds. Fly maggots in poultry manure eat tapeworm and ascarid eggs. The immature larvae are retained in the gut when the maggots become mature flies. If infected flies are eaten by the birds, the birds are exposed to the parasites. In addition, flies carry ascarid eggs and eggs of other nematodes on their bodies as they fly from manure to bird pens, feed, and/or water.

Sanitation is the key to house-fly control. Without sanitation, chemical control and other control efforts are likely to fail. Poultry manure is the preferred environment for breeding flies, so manure management becomes the key to handling the fly problem. Try to keep fly populations under control. During the summer, clean the house weekly and spread the manure thinly. Eggs and larvae will not survive the effect of drying the manure. This will break the life cycle.

In caged breeder operations, an all-out fly-control program of regular (i.e., scheduled) insecticide applications may be necessary. Keep in mind that flies become resistant to a particular insecticide after time. For this reason, best results are obtained when a combination of formulations — such as baits, residual sprays, and larvicides — are used during the fly season. Conditions vary with each poultry operation; so fly-control programs must be "tailor-made" for maximum clout.

Dispose of dead birds daily. Promptly remove spoiled feed, broken eggs, or any material in the litter that attracts adult flies. Keep manure as dry as possible, making it less attractive to adult flies. Repair leaks in waterers and do not splash water on droppings when cleaning waterers. Keep grass and weeds near the poultry house cut close, eliminating resting areas for mature flies (helpful for mosquito control, too). In essence, a clean, neatly kept operation will have far fewer problems than one lacking such attention.

Residual insecticides are chemicals that retain toxicity and will kill flies for several weeks after application. Residual fly-control materials should not be applied to birds or to surfaces that come in contact with feed. With this limitation in mind, spray the insecticide on all fly resting surfaces. Residuals soon become nontoxic if applied to concrete or brick surfaces, and to surfaces exposed to direct sunlight. You can improve performance if you paint or whitewash such surfaces before spraying. DO NOT SPRAY insecticide mixture on Styrofoam insulation!

Baits and larvicides are effective in reducing fly numbers in some situations. These chemicals must come in direct contact with flies and maggots. A sprinkling can may be used to apply larvicides lightly and evenly over the manure. Water emulsions can be used, but they may liquidize the manure and increase fly development. Use baits carefully to keep them from the birds or accidentally contaminating the feed.

LICE

Chewing lice belong to the order Mallophaga, class Insecta. As many as 40 species of lice have been identified in barnyard flocks or on birds on range. The species important to gamebirds and poultry are head lice (*Cuclotogaster heterographa*), body lice (*Menacanthus stramineus*), shaft lice (*Menopon gallinae*), wing lice (*Lipeurus caponis*), fluff lice (*Goniocotes gallinae*), large chicken lice (*Goniodes gigas*), brown chicken lice (*Goniodes dissimilis*), large turkey lice (*Chelopistes meleagridis*), and slender turkey lice (*Oxylipeurus polytrapezius*). *M. stramineus* will infest turkeys. Sucking lice do not attack birds. Chewing lice are parasites who spend all life stages, generation after generation, on the host bird. Lice spread from bird to bird by contact. The new (receiving) host is usually the younger of the birds. Some lice will move to a different species of bird, if the opportunity presents.

LIFE CYCLE:

Lice, like all insects, have three distinct body parts — head, thorax (chest), and abdomen. Insects have three pairs of legs attached to the thorax. Lice do not have wings as do many other types of insects. The mature louse is wingless, flat-bodied, six-legged, with double claws and round head. The chewing mouth parts, located on the ventral side of the head, are prominent and serrated. The average female lays and cements from 50 to 300 eggs to the feathers of the host. Louse eggs are generally white and oval-shaped, and may be covered with fine spines. Although laid singly, the eggs may be so numerous as to form visible clusters on the fluffy feathers of heavily infested birds. Lice eggs begin to hatch within a few days but some may require as long as 2 weeks. Young nymphs (though smaller and transparent), closely resemble mature lice.

Running and feeding activity begins immediately. The nymphs pass through several molts within a few weeks, gradually assuming the coloration, form, and size of mature lice. Full-grown lice may be up to an eighth of an inch in length and body color varies from gray to yellow to black. Lice may live several months. Time from hatch to maturity is about 4 to 6 weeks, with numerous generations per year. Lice, though active throughout the year, are most abundant during the summer.

PATHOLOGY:

Bird lice feed on dry scales, feathers, or scabs on the skin. Some species ingest blood exuding from irritated areas or from emerging feathers. As lice crawl over the bird, their mouth parts and sharp claws scratch the skin. The constant irritation causes the bird to become nervous and behave abnormally, creating an unthrifty and unkempt appearance in the bird. Birds add to the damage by pecking and scratching at lice or skin irritations. Feather lice feed on the barbules. The plumage becomes dry and ruffled. Egg production in infested flocks may drop as much as 10 to 20 percent. If brooding hens are heavily infested, the hatchlings may die from the infestation.

CONTROL:

Effective control of lice requires the use of a chemical pesticide. Control procedures are much the same for all lice species. Lice are sensitive to most insecticides, but only a few insecticides are safe and approved for use on poultry.

Available pesticides are dusting powders (dust), wettable powders for sprays, and emulsion concentrates for use as sprays. The dust formulations are packaged ready-to-use, and are applied by picking up and dusting each bird individually. Hens in cages may be dusted with a power duster.

Sprays may be directed onto the birds on floors or in cages. For noncommercial and specialty flocks reared on the floor, dusting the litter and providing a square dust box (18" on a side and 4" deep) charged with the insecticide dust is a good control method. The birds will dust themselves. Currently available pesticides effective against lice include Sevin, Rabon, Malathion, Co-ral, and RaVap.

MOSQUITOES

AND MOSQUITO CONTROL

FACTS ABOUT MOSQUITOS

1. The adult female mosquito feeds on blood; for this reason, its bite may be dangerous to gamebirds and domestic poultry, and to humans and other mammals. The adult male mosquito feeds on plant juices.

2. Mosquito development involves four stages — egg, larva, pupa, and adult. The adult mosquito is a flying insect; eggs are laid and hatch in water; larval and pupal development follow. Mosquitoes do not leave the water until they become flying adults. The larval and pupal stages do not bite.

3. The mosquito's life cycle is about 6 days in summer, but longer in cool weather.

4. Eight species of mosquitoes, of five genera, may be dangerous to poultry because they can be vectors (carriers) of EEE — the EEE-type virus overwinters in eggs of these species. They are *Aedes triseriatus, A. trivittatus, A. vexans, Culex restuans, C. salinarius, C. territans, Culiseta melanura,* and *Mansonia perturbans.*

Species identification is necessary, because successful control depends on timing of treatment and the area treated. Some species are of little public health or economic importance. Control of larvae requires knowledge of where the species breeds and flight areas of the mature mosquito. It is of little use to fog, for example, when the adults are resting. It may be that good control can be achieved without the use of an insecticide.

Breeding habits and areas of the nine species are as follows:

Aedes triseriatus is a tree-hole mosquito. Larvae develop in water that is standing in tree holes. Adults do not fly far from breeding sites. *A. triseriatus* feeds on the blood of birds, humans, and other mammals.

Aedes trivittatus belongs to the flood-water group of mosquitoes. These develop in still or backwater pools created by rain or stream overflow. This mosquito ranges usually no more than a mile and a half from its "home pool," and feeds readily on humans.

Aedes vexans is likewise is a flood-water species. Its larvae can be found in rain-filled containers, puddles, and rainfed woodland pools. It has a long flight range, traveling as far as 10 miles from its breeding grounds. *Aedes vexans* feeds on birds, humans, and domestic animals, and is widely distributed in the United States.

Culex restuans breeds in pools, ditches, and other places where rain water collects. Its flight range is short (less than 3 miles). This mosquito feeds on domestic and wild birds, and occasionally bites humans.

Culex salinarius deposits eggs in many water habitats, including fresh and brackish pools and stagnant swamps. It feeds on birds, humans, and other mammals, and may range as far as 8 miles from its home pool.

Culex territans larvae develop in vegetated pools and ponds; it generally avoids foul water. This species is not known to bite humans, but feeds on amphibians and reptiles, and occasionally on birds.

Culiseta melanura breeds in acid water, such as sphagnum bogs and cedar swamps. Primarily a feeder on birds, C. *melanura* may be the most important vector of encephalitis, carrying the EEE organism from bird to bird.

Mansonia perturbans breeds in marshes and bogs. In the larval form it remains attached to submerged aquatic plants and will not be found at the water's surface. Its flight range is extensive — as long as 15 miles. Adults feed on humans.

FACTS ABOUT MOSQUITO CONTROL

1. Effective control requires survey and accurate identification of the mosquito species in the area. Skilled entomologists can identify the species from intact immature forms or from adults. Survey involves sampling suspected breeding pools for larval or pupal forms; usually by dipping and inspection. If larval or pupal forms are present, specific species identification is required. Collect mature forms with a sweep net, again taking care not to damage the specimens.

Bottle specimens in rubbing (isopropyl) or ethyl alcohol. Immature forms must first be strained or filtered from the water. Send the bottled samples to a mosquito specialist. Usually county extension offices or public health offices can suggest or provide vector-control specialists that specialize in mosquito work and can identify mosquitoes by species.

2. The female mosquito requires a blood meal before she can deposit her eggs and a pool of water to deposit them in. Rainwater collects in discarded cans and cartons, old tires, discarded tennis shoes, farm equipment, feed bins, plastic fertilizer bags, wading pools, and trench silo covers—any cavity that holds water will soon be quite acceptable

as a nursery for mosquito larvae. Cleaning up trash and getting rid of standing water is a first step to fewer mosquitoes.

Some poultry houses are screened to prevent mosquitoes from getting to the birds. On others, the rubbish collection area is sometimes roofed over to prevent rain pooling in the trash. Rubbish disposal must always be in accordance with good environmental practice — if there's an open dump within a few miles, your birds may still be within the feeding grounds of hungry migrant mosquitoes.

3. Adult mosquitoes rest on twigs and branches, and females fly about in search of blood meals and pools for egg-laying. This behavior is a factor in control programs. Any action that reduces the number of pools or increases the flight time between resting, feeding, and pools for laying eggs means, in the end, fewer eggs per female. This is why clearing out vegetation from around ponds and lakes and from areas around pens is frequently suggested as a mosquito control practice.

Although species vary somewhat in their flight habits, most rest during the day and fly to seek feeding areas and pools for egg-laying near dusk and in early evening. Fogging with insecticides to control flying mosquitoes is effective only during these hours. The most effective control programs are those directed against the immature stages, such as the elimination of breeding pools. Chemical treatment of any stream or other sizable body of water is likely to require approval of the appropriate public health and environmental protection agencies. Using a mosquito-control specialist may be a good idea, as this individual will be up-to-date on regulatory requirements as well as approved chemicals (if needed) and their correct application.

Wide-area mosquito control programs are underway in many areas, usually managed by public health or environmental protection agencies. It's a good idea to cooperate in such efforts. Payoff of a well-planned wide-area control effort usually far exceeds that achievable by individual gamebird growers. Most extension offices will know about these projects, and can provide up-to-date information about managing mosquito problems.

CHIGGER MITE

Chigger mites, *Neoschongastia americana*, are parasites of gamebirds and turkeys on open range. Dense feathered hairs usually covering mature chiggers give them a velvety appearance. The covering of feathered hairs is less dense on the larvae. The body is shaped as a figure "eight" and is often bright red. Chiggers are about 1/25 inch in length. Larvae are about 1/150-inch in length and reddish or straw-colored. Bird carcasses showing lesions caused by chiggers are graded downward when processed. Chiggers feed in clusters on the thighs, breast, undersides of the wings, and vent areas. Chigger bites produce scabby, reddish lesions that require 3 weeks to heal.

LIFE CYCLE:

Mature chiggers do not feed. Larval chiggers feed once, usually for 4 days. Some may feed as long as a month before becoming engorged with food. Chiggers normally do not burrow into the skin or suck blood. The parasitic larvae firmly attach themselves to the skin of the host, and then inject a salivary enzyme, "digesting" surrounding tissues. The "dissolved" tissue is then sucked up, as food, by the chigger. After engorgement, it drops to the ground. Adult chigger mites live in the soil; the larval mites live in soil and on vegetation. They climb up on grass and plants to reach birds.

PATHOLOGY:

The main pathology is the chigger bite. Bites leave red erythematous welts that itch, prompting the bird to scratch and damage plumage and/or skin. The injury scabs over, and must be trimmed from the body at processing, down-grading the carcass. Heavy chigger infestations reduce bird performance by decreasing growth and production.

CONTROL:

Control of chiggers on the range is aided by keeping the grass cut short and periodically dusting with sulfur or malathion. Other FDA-approved pesticides may also be used. Chiggers present the greatest problem in the late summer and fall.

Southern climates are conducive for chiggers year-around. The gamebird grower must be alert to the presence of this parasite and establish a program for its control. It may become necessary to abandon heavily infested outdoor pens.

DEPLUMING MITE

Depluming mites, *Knemidocoptes gallineae,* are related to and resemble the scaly leg mites, *K. mutans. K. gallineae* is smaller. The female is 0.3 mm in diameter. Dorsal striations form raised sculpturing. Prevalent in the spring and summer, the mites spread by direct body contact. *K. gallineae* burrow into the base of the feather shaft on the epidermis of birds, especially pheasant, pigeon, and chickens. The intense irritation causes the affected bird to pull its own feathers, hence, depluming mite.

LIFE CYCLE:

The life cycle of *Knemidocoptes gallineae* is like that of the scaly-leg mite. The mites pass the entire life cycle in the skin and feathers of the bird. Transmission or spread is bird to bird by body contact.

PATHOLOGY:

The bird is injured by disrruption of the thermo-regulation function and loss of body heat due to depluming and feather damage. Likewise with feather pulling and skin irritations, the bird is continually combating cutaneous infections. Some infested birds lose weight as well as lay fewer eggs.

Gamebirds with depluming mite feather damage are of no value for release or hunt. Heavily parasitized birds are unthrifty. Open wounds are subject to bacterial infections, many (e.g., staphylococcosis) of which become systemic. Flock mortality increases.

CONTROL:

Controlling depluming mites is difficult. Immediate isolation of affected birds and pens is recommended. Buildings should be cleaned and disinfected, as outlined for red chicken mites. Treat birds with a spray of an approved poultry pesticide (see listing, p 231). Apply the pesticide in split treatments with half the total recommended dose at each application. Implement strict biosecurity and sanitation within and between pens to prevent further spread or reintroduction of the mite on the farm.

FEATHER MITE

There are a variety of feather mites. Members of four biological families, they represent five genera of mites. Feather mites tend to be host specific. All feather mites except *Syringophilus* belong to the super family *Analgesoidae*. The quill mite, *Syringophilus hipectinatus*, lives inside the feather quill of gamebirds and poultry.

Wild birds harbor related mite species. *S. columbae* infests pigeon and *S. minor* infests house sparrow. Both are often involved with gamebirds. The female mites are elongated and measure 0.9 mm in length and 0.15 mm in width. *S. hipectinatus* has been found in golden pheasant, chickens, and turkeys from New England to the midwestern states. Other mites that damage feathers belong to five genera. *Falculifer* spp occurs between the barbules of large wing feathers of pigeons. *Freyana* are in the grooves on the underside shafts of wing feathers of turkeys. *Dermoglyphus* are inside turkey quills. *Pterolichus* are on flight and tail feathers of chickens. *Megninia* occurs on the head and legs of turkeys and chickens. Others of this genus deplume the neck and body areas of pigeons.

LIFE CYCLE:

Mites are members of the spider family. The eggs hatch into nymphs. Nymphs undergo a series of molts to become adults. The cycle of development from egg to sexually mature feather mites for *Syringophylus* is 38 to 41 days. Female mites hatch from eggs laid by fertilized female mites. Male mites hatch from eggs deposited by nonfertilized females. Life cycles of other genera of mites are very similar. Many of the mites spend the entire life cycle without leaving the host.

PATHOLOGY:

The quill mites cause partial to complete loss of feathers. The remaining quill stumps contain a powdery material in which mites can be detected under low power magnification. Diagnosis is based on the demonstration and identification of the respective feather mite. Other feather mites damage the feathers. In bird species raised for their plumage, feather mites become a serious economical factor.

Gamebirds with feather mites are not suitable for release on hunting preserves. Economic damage in domestic poultry can be enumerated as loss of eggs, malnutrition, dermatitis, and loss of feathers. Birds in mite-infested areas develop crust-like lesions on comb, wattles, and legs.

CONTROL:

There is no method of control for the quill mite. The present option involves total depopulation of the flock, secure disposal of carcasses, followed by thorough C& D of premises. An application of a mitacidal pesticide after C& D is recommended.

Control of other feather mites would follow the combined programs for red mite and northern fowl mite. See table, p 231,for FDA- and EPA-approved pesticides for use on poultry or in poultry houses. Carbaryl, coumaphos, and malathion are among the pesticides approved as poultry pest -control chemicals.

NORTHERN FOWL MITE

The northern fowl mite, *Ornithonyssus sylviarum*, is the most common and economically most important of the poultry mites. The northern fowl mite infests gamebirds, especially pheasants, chickens, and turkeys. Mites are a problem in all poultry production areas in the United States, and a serious pest throughout the temperate zones of other countries. These mites are common parasites in caged-bird complexes and birds on range.

The northern fowl mite has been reported on many bird species and may be introduced to gamebird and poultry operations by English sparrows. It is sometimes mistaken for the red chicken mite, but, unlike the red mite, the northern mite can be found on birds in the day time as well as night. It can be spotted on the bird by parting the feathers about the vent. Caretakers often see mites on the eggs.

LIFE CYCLE:

The life cycle of the northern mite requires less than a week. Eggs are laid on the feathers and hatch within 24 hours. The entire life cycle is spent on the host; growth from egg through nymphal stages to maturity is completed in about 4 days. Because of this short time from hatch to maturity, infestations can reach astronomical numbers in a relatively short time. Gamebird growers can estimate infestation levels by blowing the feathers and counting the mites seen. If five are seen, the bird may be carrying from 100 to 300 mites. If six are seen, 300 to 1000 are likely to be present; seven, 1000 to 3000; eight, 3000 to 10,000; nine, 10,000 to 32,000 or so. Northern fowl mite infestations may dwindle some in the summer, but are more severe in winter. For the red mite, the reverse is true. Away from its avian host, the northern fowl mite may survive 3 to 4 weeks.

PATHOLOGY:

Northern fowl mites are blood feeders. Anemia occurs in heavily parasitized birds, reducing efficiency, production, and ability to withstand and overcome diseases. Scabby areas blemish the skin of market birds, reducing their value. Egg production falls off in laying flocks. Breeding males produce less semen. If infestations incur 200,000 or more mite bites, a fatal anemic condition can be expected. Interference with the bird's immune response is probably a key factor.

Mite-stressed birds lose weight, have pink combs, and feathers soiled by mite excrement. Feathers around the vent area become black. The northern fowl mite is capable, after feeding on birds infected with avian viruses, of harboring the virus for some time. This species has not, however, been shown to be a causative factor in serious viral epidemics.

CONTROL:

The first and perhaps most important step in parasite control is accurate identification of the parasite. The adult northern fowl mite measures about 1/26 in in length. Accurate identification requires examination under magnification. As with the red mite, the elliptical anal plate, located on the long axis of the mite, is the distinguishing characteristic. The anal pore is at the top of the anal plate.

Total mite control requires the use of chemical pesticides. Mites are more resistant than lice, so a rotation of pesticides used may be necessary. Pesticides for the northern fowl mite must be applied to the bird as wettable powder or emulsion concentrate sprays or as dust. For small, floor-reared flocks, the application of a dust may be effective — treat the bird and the litter and provide dust boxes. When spraying floor birds, bunch the birds in a corner, then direct the spray toward their vent areas; with caged birds, spray up through the bottom of the cage. Entomologists recommend spraying at least twice initially, applying half-doses about 30 minutes apart. This practice will provide better feather penetration of the pesticide.

Pesticides, besides those approved for lice control, include Atroban, Ectiban, Overtime, Insectrin, and Permectrin II. These pesticides are trademarked, and are listed here by their trade names. Avoid illegal use or misuse of the product by paying careful attention to label instructions. Between flocks, clean, disinfect, fumigate and/or spray the building with a pesticide.

RED MITE

The red mite, *Dermanyssus gallinae*, is a common external parasite in poultry that is more prevalent in small noncommercial flocks than in large commercial flocks. Husbandry and management of the respective operations probably account for this difference in occurrence. Other names for the red mite are chicken mite, gray mite, and roost mite. The red mite is found worldwide and is a particular problem in warmer temperate climates. Domestically, the mite is more prevalent in poultry houses equipped with roosts. Chickens are the preferred host, but gamebirds, turkeys, pigeons, canaries, and wild birds are infested, too. Human dwellings have been known to become infested from sparrows that nest beneath the eaves of the house or building.

LIFE CYCLE:

The red mite runs rapidly on the skin and feathers. It is a true mite and therefore an arachnid, a member of the spider family. Mites have two major body parts — the cephalothorax and abdomen. Four pairs of legs attach to the abdomen. Red mites are blood-feeders; so after feeding, the mite is red. This mite lives in secluded cracks and crevices on the roost, walls, ceiling, and floors of poultry houses. They are nocturnal feeders; therefore, usually not found on the bird during the day. Setting hens may be attacked during the day. Infestation may go undetected unless the birds are examined at night. If suspected, mites can be found by examining secluded hiding areas in the house, looking for masses of mites, mite eggs, and excrement deposits that are black and white in these places.

Red mites feed during two nymphal stages and several times as adults. Females require a blood meal before laying eggs. The female begins laying her eggs the the day after she feeds. Within 2 to 3 days the eggs hatch into nonfeeding six-legged larval mites. Larvae molt in 1 to 2 days. Nymphs, after the first molt, have eight legs and begin to feed. Under favorable conditions, the life cycle requires 10 days which makes possible many generations per year. Infestation increases through the spring, summer, and fall. In winter, the red mite is inactive except in heated poultry houses. In empty houses, the mites remain dormant for 4 to 5 months in the summer and even longer in winter.

PATHOLOGY:

The adult mite is about 1/35-inch long. Red mites feed on blood; so heavy infestations cause birds to become anemic, droopy, and weak with pale combs and wattles. Feed efficiency and egg production is reduced. Young hatchlings and setting hens may die from blood loss.

Birds in production may refuse to lay in infested nests. This is an indication that the poultry house should be examined for mites. The red mite has been reported to transmit fowl cholera and the fowl spirochete *Borrelia anserina*.

CONTROL:

Accurate identification of the species is the first step in control. This is done by examining several of the mites under the microscope. Red mite must be differentiated from the northern fowl mite. The identifying feature or key to red mite identification is the anal plate on the ventrocaudal region of the mite's body. The anal plate is large and shield-shaped, and the anal opening is near its caudal end.

Once diagnosis is confirmed, treat the areas of the poultry house where the mites hide. Effective control requires thorough C&D of the building, followed by one or more applications of an approved poultry miticide. Treat wooden roosts with a carbolenium compound. If all else fails, the building may have to be rested for a long period or abandoned for poultry housing.

SCALY LEG MITE

The scaly leg mite, *Knemidocoptes mutans*, seldom causes trouble in well-managed commercial flocks. These eight-legged mites burrow under the scales on the feet and lower legs of domestic and wild birds, causing an itch and irritation. Scales on the legs become elevated and are easily detached. Scabs form about them, and a fine white dust sifts from beneath them. Lymph and blood exude from the lesions, and red blotches form on the legs. Unless treated, the legs and feet become distorted, interfering with joint flexion and causing lameness. Severe infestations may cause the loss of one or more toes, loss of appetite, drop in egg production, weight loss, and death.

LIFE CYCLE:

Female scaly leg mites begin depositing eggs soon after they burrow under the scales and continue to oviposit for about 2 months. Eggs hatch in about 5 days; the six-legged larvae soon molt to eight-legged nymphal stages and into mature males and immature females. Maturity of the female occurs shortly after she is fertilized, and egg laying begins. The life cycle is complete in approximately 2 weeks. The pale gray eight-legged adults are up to 1/100 inch across, nearly circular in outline, and can be seen only with magnification. The same mite infests psittacine birds, where owners refer to it as the "Face and Leg Mite."

PATHOLOGY:

Lesions are produced on unfeathered portions of the host's legs and feet. Tunnels are bored into the skin causing proliferation of the epithelium and formation of scales and crusts. Affected birds may become crippled if infestation is severe and untreated. In pet cage birds, lesions appear on the beak around the cere. The facial form causes enlargement and distortion of the beak.

CONTROL:

Control is achieved by dipping the bird (up to the hock, feet and shanks) in motor oil, diesel oil, or kerosene. For psittacine birds, mix pesticide into medicinal oil and apply topically to face, feet, and legs. Repeat once or twice at weekly intervals. Houses should be frequently cleaned and sprayed with FDA- approved pesticide.

FOWL TICK

The fowl tick, *Argas persicus*, is also called the blue bug or chicken tick. Fowl tick is a pest of gamebirds and poultry, and is the only tick that attacks birds. Sucking of blood by fowl ticks causes birds to be unthrifty, lose weight, and lay fewer eggs. Birds infested with ticks show weakness in the legs, droopiness of the wings, and loss of appetite. In chicks, loss of blood can cause death. The fowl tick transmits fowl spirochetosis, a fatal disease to many birds.

LIFE CYCLE:

Mature fowl ticks are flat, leathery, eight-legged, thin-bodied, egg-shaped, reddish to blue-black, and 1/4 to 1/2 inch long. The six-legged larvae are 1/10 inch long and dark blue or purplish. The non-engorged nymphal ticks are gray with eight legs. There are usually two and sometimes three nymphal stages. Mature fowl ticks deposit eggs in cracks and rough places of poultry houses or roosting areas.

When the tick eggs hatch, the young larvae attach themselves to birds to suck blood for about a week. After engorgement, ticks drop off to seek hiding places to molt. Nymphs usually feed on the host at night or in subdued light in which they engorge themselves with blood for 30 to 60 minutes before leaving the host. The entire life cycle requires a minimum of 30 to 40 days if food and temperature are suitable, but frequently the time is much longer. Once established in poultry facilities, fowl ticks are difficult to control. Adult ticks can live as long as 2 years without feeding, so short-time "resting" of housing will not control this parasite.

PATHOLOGY:

The fowl tick is capable of transmitting diseases. The disease associated with the tick is *Borrelia anserina*, a spirochete that is highly infectious to all birds. Diseases less-often spread or introduced by infected ticks are pullorum and fowl cholera. Direct pathological effects are anemia (from loss of blood) and tick paralysis, afebrile motor paralysis. Clinical signs may be confused with botulism, Marek's disease, Newcastle disease, and avian influenza.

CONTROL:

Control requires treatment of premises to eliminate fowl ticks from hiding places. Application of approved pesticides upon completion of C&D is recommended. High-pressure spraying of the building with a 3% malathion gives some measure of tick control. To completely destroy the ticks, it may be necessary to fumigate the faciLity with formaldehyde.

Larval ticks can be controlled by dipping birds into 0.5 percent malathion. Replacement birds should be free of ticks. Even then, treat replacement birds with pesticides before housing. Regular searches for ticks on birds and in the building is a part of an ongoing tick-monitoring program.

GROWER'S REFERENCE

ON

GAMEBIRD HEALTH

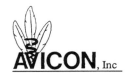

AVICON, Inc

NUTRITIONAL DISEASES

OVERVIEW

Gamebirds require approximately 40 essential nutrients. Most of these are present in the grains and other feedstuffs that form the bird's daily ration. Birds in high production may require diets carefully supplemented with extra nutrients, including additional minerals and vitamins.

Some nutrients are used in minute amounts and may be toxic if ingested in larger amounts. Excess trace nutrients create health problems potentially as serious and costly as a disease. Some trace nutrients must be ingested in relatively small quantities in order to support proper metabolism. For example, the ratio of calcium to phosphorus should be about two to one. An excess of either may interfere with the ability of the bird to absorb and metabolize both minerals.

Most manufacturers of commercial poultry feeds try to provide all essential nutrients, including minerals and vitamins. Dietary adjustments may be required in periods of high stress such as a disease outbreak or severe environmental conditions. If nutritional problems are present, the bird tends to become more susceptible to disease. Thus, nutrition management is as important as biosecurity in successful gamebird production.

VITAMIN A DEFICIENCY

Vitamin **A** is an essential nutrient for young poultry. Poultry of all ages will suffer from prolonged deficiency of vitamin **A**. If the starter ration is markedly deficient in vitamin **A**, chicks become stunted and growth rates decline rapidly after 3 weeks. The birds become unthrifty and droopy; feathers are ruffled. As effects of the deficiency advance, nasal discharges develop, the eyes swell, and pustules with a sticky exudate form in the mouth and esophagus. Unless the deficiency is corrected, mortality may reach 100 percent.

Vitamin **A** deficiency is called "Nutritional Roup."

Gamebirds and poults are more severely affected than chicks. In mature birds, inadequate vitamin **A** causes a drop in production and reduced hatchability of fertile eggs. Nutritional roup is characterized by keratinization that indicates damaged epithelial tissues. Vitamin **A** has been shown to be the keeper of epithelium. Epithelial tissues, the basic components of the skin, mucus membranes, and glands, are the first line of defense against infection for the bird. Vitamin **A** is required for normal individual growth and tissue repair, as well as for normal bone development.

CLINICAL SIGNS:

The clinical signs of keratinization are squamous epithelial cell metaplasia, i.e., patchy thickening on epithelial surfaces. Other clinical signs of nutritional roup include whitish pustules and sticky exudates on epithelial surfaces. These lesions are most obvious on the linings of the mouth, nasal passages, pharynx, and esophagus.

PATHOLOGY:

Lesions may include urate deposits in the kidneys, ureters, cloaca, and bursa of Fabricius. Vitamin **A** deficiency lesions may be subtle and hard to recognize in mild cases, in contrast to the typical lesions of severe nutritional roup syndrome. If detected before severe kidney damage occurs, the condition is reversible by correcting the vitamin **A** deficiency. Diagnostic clues are history, symptoms, lesions, and absence of infections.

CONTROL:

Control is achieved by correcting the deficiency of vitamin **A** in the ration plus 5 to 7 days' supplementation of water-dispersible vitamin **A** in the drinking water. The requirement of vitamin **A** is 15 million

IU/ton of feed for starter and breeder feeds and 12 million IU/ton of feed for grower and maintenance feeds. Sources of vitamin A include yellow corn, legumes, grasses, fish oils, and dry stabilized vitamin A supplements. Vitamin A in many feedstuffs will deteriorate over time; thus the need for a stabilized supplement. Stresses from diseases such as coccidiosis, molds, worms, and other intestinal disorders increase the need for vitamin A above the minimum requirement. Vitamin A supplementation is likewise recommended as adjunct therapy for various infections of the gastrointestinal tract.

RICKETS

Rickets is a nutritional disorder, primarily of young poultry, caused by a deficiency or imbalance of calcium, vitamin D_3, or phosphorus. This disease, characterized by abnormal skeletal development, is most readily detectable in the leg's long bones. Rickets is the disease of young poultry and osteomalacia is the disease of adult poultry.

Rickets can show a number of variations, reflecting different deficiencies or imbalances of the minerals and vitamins involved. Lesions of either calcium or vitamin D_3 rickets are alike because they are interrelated. Deficiency of either calcium or vitamin D_3 prevents sufficient calcification of bone. If calcium is lacking in the feed, it cannot be ingested and absorbed by the bird. If the vitamin D_3 is insufficient, the bird can not utilize ingested calcium, and the result is the same as a calcium deficiency. Calcium absorption is the primary dietary role of vitamin D_3 which must be present for normal calcium utilization. In vitamin D_3 and/or calcium deficiency, the leg bones are soft and springy; birds may become weak and paretic as the condition advances. When phosphorus is deficient, the leg bones are soft and rubbery and the joints tend to enlarge, but the bird does not become paralyzed. Rickets often affects poultry younger than 6 weeks.

CLINICAL SIGNS:

Rickets is the result of feeding-management errors, medication practices, and in some cases, mold or mycotoxins in the feed. Certain molds and their toxins interfere with vitamin D_3 absorption and utilization by the bird. A three- or fourfold level of vitamin D_3 is usually necessary for a margin of safety in such cases.

Calcium/vitamin D_3 rickets is seen when the vitamin is inadvertently omitted from the commercial vitamin premix or the calcium level is intentionally reduced for potentiation (reducing calcium levels to enhance antibiotic activity) of starter feeds with tetracycline antibiotics. Calcium interferes with the absorption of tetracycline by the bird; therefore, the calcium level in starter feeds may be deliberately reduced during periods of medication. In these situations the available calcium in the starter ration may be reduced to only one-fourth that actually needed by the birds. An excess of either calcium or available phosphorus in the feed can cause rickets; the ratio of calcium to phosphorus must be about 2:1 for proper metabolism.

PATHOLOGY:

Diagnosis of rickets is based on feeding history, feed analysis, and typical lesions. The epiphysial growth plate of the long bones of the leg should be examined. Calcium/vitamin D_3 rickets induces wide or abnormal epiphysis of affected long bones, and the bones are springy when checked for breaking strength. Phosphorus rickets causes soft rubbery bones; the epiphysial growth plate is normal but thin. It has been reported that rickets can be present in certain infectious conditions such as infectious bursal disease. When infectious lesions are present, additional laboratory checks should be made to confirm the disease and to differentiate it from dietary rickets.

CONTROL:

Rickets is treated by correcting problems related to the ration. It may be that the feed is moldy, or that an actual deficiency of one or more of the key trace ingredients (calcium, phosphorus, or vitamin D_3) exists. A serious overage or underage of any of these in the ration will prevent the bird from obtaining the proper ratios and avoiding rickets.The recommended levels for gamebird feeds are calcium (1.23%), phosphorus (0.55%), and vitamin D_3 (2 million IU/ton). Providing water-dispersible vitamins containing vitamin D_3 for 3 to 7 days is recommended as supplementary therapy.

PEROSIS

Perosis is caused by a deficiency of the mineral element manganese (Mn). Mn is essential, in trace amounts, for the development of normal bone, tendon, and joint cartilages in birds. In young birds, a Mn deficiency causes perosis or slipped tendon. In laying hens, a shortage of Mn will cause the bird to produce thin shelled eggs with poor hatchability of the fertile eggs. Most poultry feedstuffs are poor sources of Mn. Birds grown on wire are more susceptible to Perosis than birds reared on the floor.

CLINICAL SIGNS:

In young birds, the primary clinical signs are flattened and enlarged hocks, slippage, and lateral rotation of the Achilles tendon out of the tibial condyles. When this occurs, the shank and foot remain flexed and extended laterally from the body. The leg bones, compared to those of normal birds, tend to be shorter and thicker. In adult laying birds, the legs are not affected but egg production will drop; shells will be thinner; and embryonic death causes poor hatchability. Gamebirds require from 35 to 50 ppm of Mn in the feed to prevent perosis.

PATHOLOGY:

The primary pathological change in the growing bird is the crippling caused by the malformation of the hock joints. All joint tissues — bone, ligament, and articular cartilages — are affected. The metatarsal bone flattens, bends, and rotates. Perosis is often confused with the condition in broilers called "Twisted Leg." Bones of the leg and wing are predominant targets of this malady. Conditions in poults, ducklings, and goslings are similar to those described in chickens. Perosis is far more prevalent in chickens than in other birds because of the intensive genetic selection for birds that grow rapidly into compact heavy birds. Perosis has been reported in pheasant, grouse, quail, and sparrow, with the primary lesions affecting skeletal long bones and joints.

CONTROL:

There is no treatment for birds already affected, but a correction in the diet will prevent the development of new cases. A recommended treatment is a mineral-vitamin supplement for 3 to 5 days in the drinking water. Supplementary Mn can be added to the feed by the manufacturer. Gamebird rations should contain 66 to 85 g Mn/ton.

Starter and breeder feed should be at the higher level. The rule of thumb on perosis morbidity is that when 5 or more birds per 1000 are affected, the level of Mn in the feed should be checked. Supplemental Mn may be given in either feed or water. Most corn-soybean based poultry feed can be supplemented so that the Mn content is no less than 75 ppm. Mn content exceeding 100 ppm is wasteful.

CURLED TOE PARALYSIS

Riboflavin, or vitamin B2, is one of several B vitamins. It is also called vitamin G. Only a few natural feedstuffs contain sufficient riboflavin to meet the nutritional needs of young gamebirds and poultry.

CLINICAL SIGNS:

Toes of riboflavin-deficient chicks and poults curl medially. Other signs of riboflavin deficiency are stunting, diarrhea, and high mortality. Mortality, in young flocks on rations severely deficient in riboflavin, begins within 8 to 10 days Chicks will die before the toes begin to curl. Affected birds first rest on their hocks; a slight curling of the toes will be detectable. As the condition progresses, the birds weaken and the toes curl severely.

Toes of either or both feet may be affected. The toe curling becomes pronounced when the leg is extended. In examining young poultry for curled toe paralysis, extend the legs of the bird; with the legs in this position, affected toes will curl medially toward the other foot. Other signs are stunting, diarrhea, high mortality, and poor feather growth. Wing feathers will be extra-long. Poults develop dermatitis; the vent becomes encrusted; by day 17, growth is retarded, by day 21 mortality begins. Ducklings have diarrhea and growth is stunted or stops.

PATHOLOGY:

Toe curling, especially in turkeys, seems to be quite common in birds brooded with infrared brooders. In flocks brooded with infrared, the condition is neither preventable nor is it correctable by vitamin supplementation. Riboflavin deficiency in young birds produces changes in peripheral nerve trunks. Nerves hypertrophy (enlarge) followed by degenerative changes in the myelin covering. The thymus becomes congested and atrophied. Leg muscles atrophy and become flabby; birds sit on hocks; the wings droop as though the bird can not hold them in a normal position; and the skin is dry and scaly.

Adult birds show a drop in production and hatchability; embryos are stunted and endematous. Surviving chicks will have swollen sciatic and brachial nerves that are four to five times normal diameter. Histologically, the nerve changes involve the myelin sheath. Other lesions include thymus atrophy, and pancreatic and duodenal abnormalities that are associated with the diarrheic phase of the syndrome.

CONTROL:

If more than 5 in 1000 birds show evidence of true curled toe paralysis, the ration should be supplemented with riboflavin. This vitamin is usually included when mixing commercial starter feeds for young poultry. Gamebird rations should contain riboflavin [8 to 10 g/ton], with starter and breeder rations at the higher range. Water-soluble multiple vitamins are available and can be administered in the drinking water. If curled toe paralysis is suspected, check the ration formulation. Supplemental riboflavin in the feed is the best defense against this costly paralysis.

CHICK DERMATITIS

Chick dermatitis is caused by a deficiency of pantothenic acid, a B-complex vitamin. Pantothenic acid is a component of coenzme A, which functions in formation of citric acid (vitamin C), synthesis of fatty acids, oxidation of keto acids, and acetylation of choline plus other minor metabolic reactions.

Although most avian feedstuffs are good sources of pantothenic acid, cereal diets high in meat and fish meal may be deficient. Kiln-dried corn tends to have a lesser amount of pantothenic acid since the vitamin is destroyed by heat in the drying process. Poults are more sensitive than chicks to chick dermatitis with quail being more susceptible than other gamebird species.

CLINICAL SIGNS:

Chick dermatitis is an inflammation of the unfeathered parts of young gamebirds and poultry. Early signs of chick dermatitis are ruffled feathers, unthrifty appearance, crusty scab-like lesions at the corners of the mouth and margins of the eyes and around the vent. Eyelids frequently stick together. Cracks appear on the skin on top of the toes, between the toes, and on bottoms of the feet.

PATHOLOGY:

This vitamin functions in conjunction with other B vitamins. Pantothenic acid deficiency in adult birds causes a reduction in egg production, with weakened hatchlings. In affected birds, lesions of the spinal cord are characterized by myelin-degeneration of medullated fibers. Myelin degeneration may be found in all portions of the spinal cord down to the lumbar region. Atrophy of the thymus, fatty liver, nephritis, and atrophy of the spleen have also been reported.

Chicks are emaciated. Eyelid margins are granulated and stuck together with the exudates. There is a sloughing of keratinized epithelium, noticeable between the toes and on the bottom of the feet. When birds are necropsied, pustules are found at lesion sites. Histologically, there is pronounced lymphocytic necrosis and lymphoid depletion in the bursa of Fabricius, thymus, and spleen.

CONTROL:

Administer supplemental pantothenic acid in the drinking water for 5 to 7 days. Gamebird rations should contain calcium pantothenate [14 to 18 g/ton]. Simultaneously correct deficiencies in the feed.

ENCEPHALOMALACIA

Encephalomalacia is caused by a vitamin E deficiency. Vitamin E is fat soluble and fumctions metabolically as an antioxidant. Feed substances protected by vitamin E are the essential fatty acids and other unsaturated fatty acids such as vitamins A, D3, K, carotene, and xanthophylls.

Selenium, a trace mineral that works synergistically with vitamin E, has been shown to prevent or to cure exudative diathesis (vitamin E deficiency) in chickens. Selenium is required at the 0.1 to 0.4 ppm level to prevent myopathies of the heart and gizzard muscles. Vitamin E plays a multiple role in avian nutrition.

CLINICAL SIGNS:

No outward signs occur in mature poultry that have received low levels of vitamin E. However hatchability of fertile eggs is reduced. Embryos die as early as the fourth day of incubation. Turkey embryos develop bilateral cataracts. In older males, testicular degeneration occurs with prolonged vitamin E deficiency.

Signs of encephalomalacia are incoordination, prostration, legs stretched out behind, toes flexed, retraction of heads, and death. Another manifestation is exudative diathesis in semimature birds, especially chickens. A third form is muscular dystrophy (White Muscle disease), characterized by muscle degeneration. WMD is more prevalent in gamebirds and turkeys since they do not exhibit the exudative diathesis. Skeletal muscle, heart, and gizzard are most often affected.

PATHOLOGY:

Following is the pathology of three manifestations of vitamin E deficiency in young birds :

Encephalomalacia, commonly called "crazy chick disease," is characterized in the chick by incoordination, staggering, stumbling, and paralysis. Lesions are confined to the brain, where the cerebellum (coordination center) degenerates. Nerve tissues in the cerebellum are damaged by toxic peroxides, formed during digestion, that break down the fat components of tissue cell membranes and nerve track substances. Vitamin E in the ration acts as an antioxidant that neutralizes toxic peroxides. A presumptive diagnosis may be based on history, clinical signs, absence of gross lesions, and degeneration of the cerebellum. Confirmation requires laboratory examination of the brain tissues.

Exudative Diathesis is characterized by a severe edema produced by increased capillary permeability. The early signs, ruffled feathers and morbidity, usually occur when the birds are between 5 and 8 weeks of age. The edema produces a weeping of the skin, often seen beneath the wings and on inner surfaces of the thighs. Scabs form and the tissues become gangrenous. Exudative diathesis is not a simple vitamin E deficiency. It is accompanied by selenium deficiency, but can be alleviated by correction of either of the deficiencies. Rations of corn and soybeans are sometimes low in selenium and may lead to exudative diathesis in the flock. Vitamin E is essential to assure healthy progeny.

Nutritional Muscular Dystrophy is characterized by a degeneration of muscle fibers in the breast and leg. The condition is rare in chicks under normal management because it occurs only when the ration is deficient in vitamin E and cystine or other sulfur-containing amino acids.

CONTROL:

Birds afflicted with encephalomalacia cannot be cured, but treatment of the flock with Vitamin E will prevent new cases. Preventive measures include supportive therapy and additional Vitamin E in the feed by mixing in a suitable antioxidant.

Exudative Diathesis is not a simple Vitamin E deficiency. It is accompanied by a selenium deficiency. Inorganic selenium can prevent Exudative Diathesis. When rations from corn and soybeans are low in selenium, correction of selenium as well as Vitamin E will alleviate the problem.

Nutritional Muscular Dystrophy is controlled in hatchlings by assuring adequate vitamin E in breeder rations, essential for good hatchability and vigorous progeny. Breeder feed must be fortified with vitamin E and cystine amino acid. Grower and maintenance diets for gamebirds should include a minimum of 20,000 IU of vitamin E/ton of feed. Starter and breeder diets should contain 25,000 IU/ton. The amino acid, cystine, can prevent NMD.

VITAMIN K DEFICIENCY

Vitamin **K** is a fat-soluble vitamin whose primary function is for the synthesis of prothrombin, the clotting substance of the blood. Without vitamin **K**, an abnormal prothrombin is manufactured by the liver. A deficiency of vitamin **K** and ultimately prothrombin prolongs blood-clotting time that often results in death from hemorrhage from a bruise or injury. Alfalfa meal in poultry feeds is a rich natural source of vitamins **K** and **E**. With current feed manufacturing practices, there is less vitamin **K** in soybean meal, other seed meals, and fish meals. Currently most commercial feeds are supplemented with the synthetic vitamin **K**, menadione.

CLINICAL SIGNS:

Vitamin **K** deficiency is more frequently seen in 2- to 3- week-old gamebirds and poultry. In vitamin **K**-deficient birds, the blood clotting time begins to increase after 5 to 10 days and by 12 to 14 days, hemorrhages occur spontaneously in any part of the body. A number of stress factors (coccidiosis, intestinal parasites, and toxic reaction of sulfa drugs, dicumarol, and warfarin) increase the requirement for vitamin **K**. Toxins prevent the metabolism of vitamin **K**. Clinical signs are young birds dead from hemorrhaging. Outwardly, the birds appear normal but unclotted blood is found when necropsied. The diagnostic judgment must consider the circumstances of the case such as use of rodent poisons, heavy medication with sulfa drugs, and/or feeds deficient in vitamin **K**.

PATHOLOGY:

Young birds are anemic and often exhibit hypoplastic bone marrow. Although blood-clotting time is rather accurate, determining prothrombin time (a laboratory procedure) may be more accurate. Extensive and fatal hemorrhages will be the primary pathology in vitamin **K**-deficient birds. The problem is usually confined to a specific flock unless management practices are such that multiple flocks become subject to the same predisposition. as could be the case if all birds received the same feed from the same delivery, wide use of anti-**K** rodent poisons, or heavy prolonged use of sulfa drugs. Large hemorrhages appear on breast, legs, wings, and in the abdomen. Vitamin **K**-deficient breeder rations may be the cause of increased embryo mortality if the dead embryos are hemorrhagic.

CONTROL:

Vitamin K-deficient hatchlings respond rapidly to treatment with supplemental vitamin K. Within 4 to 6 hours after vitamin K is administered to deficient chicks, the blood clotting time returns to normal. Recovery from anemia and healing of bruises and hemorrhages requires several days. The inclusion of menadione at 1.5 mg/lb of feed is an effective and common practice in the manufacture of poultry feeds. The menadione rate can be doubled in flocks with symptoms of vitamin K deficiency. Other disease and environmental stress may indicate the need for higher menadione levels in the feed. If in doubt, consult a poultry nutritionist or a feed manufacturer for recommended levels of vitamin K in gamebird diets.

FOLIC ACID

Folic acid, or Folacin, an essential trace nutrient belonging to the **B**-vitamin complex , is a nitrogenous acid found in plant foliage. Folic acid is functional in metabolic enzyme systems and is important in the metabolization of choline, methionine, and thiamin. It is also essential for nucleic acid in tissue-cell multiplication. In recent studies, folic acid deficiency was found to occur in hatchlings under field conditions that previously had been considered unlikely. Alfalfa leaf meal is added as a source of folic acid in poultry rations.

CLINICAL SIGNS:

In young chicks, the prevalent signs are retarded growth, poor feather formation, and death. In colored breeds, there is depigmentation of the feathers. Folic acid along with lysine, copper, and iron is required for feather pigmentation and prevention of agranulocyotosis, a form of macrocytic anemia. Breeders on a ration deficient in folic acid produce anemic hatchlings that show lateral paralysis or muscle weakness. Poults will also develop cervical paralysis; the necks are extended and the birds appear to gaze downward. Egg production and hatchability are reduced. Folic acid-deficient embryos show a bending of the tibiotarsus, mandibular defects, syndactylism (webfeet), and hemorrhages.

PATHOLOGY:

The pathological effect of folic acid deficiency is reflected only in the embryos and hatchlings; therefore, the diagnosis of folic acid deficiency in adult breeder birds is ascertained by the changes found in the hatchlings. Folic acid is essential for normal formation and growth of various tissues, especially blood, bone, and feathers. Folic acid functions in metabolic symbiosis with lysine, copper, iron, vitamin B_{12}, and choline in enzyme systems for normal tissue formation. The anemia is caused by the lack of blast-cell formation for erythrocytes (RBCs) in the bone marrow. Similar incomplete metabolic processes occur to produce the deformed embryos and feather pigmentation. Mild folic acid deficiency in hatchlings is reversible but the skeletal deformities are irreversible.

CONTROL:

Mild signs of folic acid deficiencies — such as weakness, paralysis, and feather depigmentation — are responsive to folic acid therapy administered via feed or drinking water. Long-term control requires correction of the imbalance or absence of folic acid in the feed of breeder birds. All starter feeds essential for chick growth and vigor should be fortified with folic acid as well as other vitamins and trace minerals. Since there is a 3- to 4-week delay in new hatches from breeders on a folic acid-deficient diet, it takes three to four hatches after the diet is corrected before the problem will be corrected. Grower and maintenance diets should contain 1,000 mg/ton of feed and starter and breeder rations should contain 1,500 mg/ton of feed.

NIACIN DEFICIENCY

Niacin, nicotinic acid, is a component in two important co-enzymes extensively involved in the metabolism of carbohydrates, fats, and protein. The role is in the metabolic reactions that furnish energy.

Evidence shows that birds can synthesize niacin, but at a rate too slow for optimum growth. Most poultry nutritionists claim that niacin deficiency does not occur in birds unless the precursor "Tryptophan" is lacking. Niacin deficiency has been observed in young poultry fed certain practical diets. Shortcomings in corn-soy rations are easily corrected by the addition of supplemental niacin.

The niacin requirement for waterfowl, turkeys, and gamebirds is much higher than that for chickens. Much of the niacin in poultry feeds is digestibly unavailable to young poultry. Adult birds more readily synthesize niacin.

CLINICAL SIGNS:

Retarded growth may be the only sign displayed by birds with border-line niacin deficiencies. Some of the young birds may develop leg disorders similar to perosis. The main difference between niacin-deficient leg problems and perosis is that the Achilles tendon rarely slips out of the condyles. Niacin and vitamin E are required to prevent leg disorders in poults. Baby waterfowl develop leg abnormalities considered to be perosis and bowed legs. Adult laying birds on a niacin-deficient ration will lose weight, egg production will decrease, and hatchability of fertile eggs will drop.

Other signs of niacin deficiency include inflammation of the mouth, diarrhea, and poor feathering. Hock disorders and mouth lesions are more prevalent in baby waterfowl.

PATHOLOGY:

The primary pathological lesions are the permanent malformations of the legs and hocks. These lesions do not respond to treatment. On the other hand, mouth lesions and poor feathering can be reversed by correcting the niacin shortage. Dietary correction reduces the inflammation of the mouth and poor feathers are replaced during regular molting.

There is evidence that implicates a niacin deficiency in fowl hysteria of birds. In fowl hysteria, niacin dietary supplement is prescribed as a part of the treatment. Niacin provides a calming effect on birds with hysteria.

CONTROL:

Niacin deficiency in gamebirds and poultry is prevented by supplementing the ration with niacin [20 mg/lb, 40 g/ton] in the feed; however, some nutritionists prescribe, for safety factors, two to two and one-half times that amount. Waterfowl do well on feeds containing niacin at 40 mg/lb.

It is best that the ration provide ample niacin. In this way, there is no need that the bird synthesize the vitamin from tryptophan. Consult a poultry nutritionist for current recommended levels of niacin for gamebird feeds. Always insist on a feed that meets the minimum daily requirements for each of the essential vitamins and trace minerals.

THIAMIN DEFICIENCY

Polyneuritis is a condition in poultry caused by a thiamin deficiency. Thiamin is also known as a vitamin B_1 and is converted in the body to an active form of thiamin phosphate that is functional in carbohydrate (energy) metabolism. Deficiency of vitamin B_1 leads to loss of appetite, anorexia, polyneuritis, and death.

CLINICAL SIGNS:

Birds with a thiamin (vitamin B_1) deficiency are excitable and flighty. Vitamin B_1 deficiency reduces the appetite, and affected birds go off feed. Injections of vitamin B_1 will reverse these symptoms. With prolonged deficiency, however, nerve degeneration causes nonreversible lameness and muscle paralysis. Gross overuse of the coccidiostat Amprolium can produce a temporary vitamin B_1 deficiency, but the symptoms and ill effects can be corrected by adding thiamin to drinking water or feed or by removing amprolium from the ration.

PATHOLOGY:

Adult birds show bluish combs and facial tissues. As the deficiency progresses, muscle paralysis sets in, beginning with the flexor muscle of the toes and progressing to the extensor muscle of the legs, wings and neck. Affected birds characteristically sit on flexed legs with head drawn back in a 'star-gazing' position. Body balance is lost and birds become recumbent. Adrenal glands enlarge; epinephrine levels increase; and genital organs, stomach, and intestine atrophy as death approaches. A high percentage of the flock can be affected.

CONTROL:

Amprolium, similar in structure to vitamin B_1, competes with the vitamin for biochemical use. Check the feed for its Amprolium level and correct if feed has excessive amounts. Most cereal grains are high in thiamin so the deficiency is not common. If deficiency is severe, individual birds must be injected with vitamin B_1 to restore appetite (thiamin stimulates the birds to eat). Since the natural feed ingredients are rich in thiamin, supplemental thiamin is not included in premixes; but vitamin B_1 is included in soluble poultry vitamin supplements to provide a safe and simple way to counteract temporary deficiencies.

BIOTIN DEFICIENCY

Biotin is a co-factor in carboxylatin (acidification) and decarboxylation reactions in the fixation of carbon dioxide. These metabolic digestive reactions are important in the growth (anabolic) process in formation of new tissue. An essential component of protein metabolism, biotin is an integral substance in muscle growth and is essential for embryonic development. In hatchlings, this **B** vitamin aids in the prevention of perosis and foot-pad dermatitis. In adult birds, it prevents fatty liver and kidney disorder.

Corn is a rich source of biotin. Some other cereal grains, however, are poor sources, and deficiencies are more prevalent in birds on diets high in wheat and barley. Other biotin sources include yeast, liver, molasses, and green leafy plants. Biotin levels in some feeds may be inadequate for the birds; however biotin is included in premixes and can be added to assure a balanced ration.

CLINICAL SIGNS:

Embryonic death in eggs of affected breeder birds. Embryos exhibit the physical deformities of parrot beak, abnormal cartilage formation, and syndactylism (web foot). Other embryonic lesions include shortened, twisted legs and shortened wing, skull, and scapula.

Embryonic deaths increase during the first and last weeks of incubation. In young birds, typical signs include broken flight feathers, soft long bones of the leg, dermatitis of the foot pads, and scab formations at the corners of the mouth and margins of the eye lids. Young birds also exhibit deformity of the tibia (the tibia is shortened), high bone density, and abnormal pattern of bone modeling. In biotin-deficient birds, the medial mid-diaphysial cortex is thicker than the lateral side. Recent research suggests that biotin is involved in "Sudden Death" syndrome in broilers and other young birds.

PATHOLOGY:

The pathological lesions associated with biotin deficiency are its effect on the health of the skin and formation of the bones. The growing birds' dermatitis and defective feathers are more obvious and are associated with the foot pad, mouth, and eye lesions.

Also, biotin bone deformity must be considered in nonmanganese-responsive perosis. Many hatchlings from biotin-deficient breeders hatch as anomalies. Most effects of biotin deficiency are not reversible; therefore, early diagnosis and treatment will prevent the development of new cases within the brood or flock.

CONTROL:

Factors that increase the biotin requirement in the diet include rancid fat in the ration, enteric infections, and hatching from eggs of breeders on a biotin-deficient ration. One research worker reported that biotin supplementation via feed or water would prevent signs of the deficiency.

Gamebird starter rations should be fortified with synthetic biotin [100 to 150 mg/ton]; likewise [100 mg/ton] for grower and maintenance rations. Biotin from natural sources is expensive and/or difficult to obtain. Certain antibiotics administered in the feed spare the need for biotin by enhancing the intestinal microflora. Biotin supplements from dried brewers' yeast and synthetic biotin are effective in either feed or water.

A logical correction for suspected trace-nutrient deficiency is the administration of biotin-containing multiple vitamins in the drinking water for 3 to 5 days. Also, check and correct the biotin level in the feed ration.

CHOLINE DEFICIENCY

Choline, a vitamin present in many animal and some plant tissues, can be synthetically produced. Choline is a component of certain enzymes that are essential for various metabolic functions. Choline is present in acetylcholine and phospholipids and acts as a methyl source in the body's synthesis of methionine and other amino acids.

Choline has several physiological functions in birds. In part, it has a role in the prevention of perosis as well as the synthesis of transport lipids. Perosis-like lesions develop in poultry suffering from choline-deficient diets, even when manganese, biotin, and niacin amounts are adequate.

Maximum egg production, high hatchability, and the prevention of the fatty liver syndrome all require choline. Practical corn-soy rations may provide choline or components for synthesis by the bird. Feed ingredients rich in choline are soybean meal, wheat bran, and wheat middlings. Other supplemental sources are brewers' grains, fish meal, liver meal, distillers' solubles, and yeast.

CLINICAL SIGNS:

The initial sign of choline deficiency is poor growth and perosis, followed (in prolonged deficiency) by pathognomonic signs. Young turkeys have a higher requirement for choline than most gamebirds or chickens. Perosis is first characterized by pin-point hemorrhages and puffiness of affected joints and is caused by the flattening and rotation of the bone of the hock (i.e., tibiometatarsal) joint. The metatarsus twists and bends out of alignment with the tibia, crippling the bird.

Fatty liver syndrome is a common sign of choline deficiency in table-egg chicken strains. When pullets are grown on high choline diets and then, as hens, receive a choline-deficient diet, the percentage of fat in the liver increases. The explanation is that normal mature birds can synthesize choline but will not develop the ability to do so if maintained on high-choline grower diets.

PATHOLOGY:

Pathological changes in choline-deficient birds include leg crippling, fatty liver disorders, and generally poor growth. Choline is an essential nutrient for normal development of bone and soft tissue. When deficient, all body tissues fail to develop normally, and the cartilage of the articular joint is damaged.

Even though the crippling in individually affected birds is permanent, the problem with growth and fatty liver syndrome ican be reversed by correcting the choline deficiency. Immature gamebirds and poultry are unable to synthesize adequate choline for their physiological needs; therefore choline must be supplemented in the diet.

CONTROL:

Choline-deficient disorders are best prevented by providing diets containing adequate levels of vitamins. The recommended levels of choline are 1,000 g/ton in starter and breeder feeds and 800 g/ton in grower and maintenance feeds. Immature birds are more severely affected than are mature gamebirds and poultry. When poor growth, fatty liver, and/or perosis are prevalent in a flock, the ration should be analyzed to assure adequate levels of essential nutrients and trace minerals.

The rule of thumb for diseases from nutritional deficiency is that when more than five birds in a thousand are affected, the probable cause is deficiency of an essential ingredient — in this case, choline. Supplementation can be made with soluble vitamins administered in the drinking water. A second approach would be to provide feed with adequate vitamins and minerals; if necessary, using a new supplier.

GROWER'S REFERENCE

ON

GAMEBIRD HEALTH

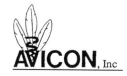

AVICON, Inc

ASCITES

Ascites is an accumulation of fluid (non-inflammatory transudate) in the abdominal cavity of gamebirds and poultry. The condition is also called water belly, right ventricular failure, pulmonary hypertension syndrome, and salt poisoning. Vitamin E and selenium deficiency or any situation that impedes or interferes with normal blood circulation can cause ascites. Fluid most frequently collects in the pericardial sac and the abdominal or peritoneal cavity and lungs. The fluid is yellowish or straw-colored and contains protein clots often seen as a gelatinous material. The causes of ascites include weakened heart muscle (cardiomyopathy), hereditary hypertension, salt poisoning, drug toxicity, anoxia during brooding, infectious omphalitis, and liver infections. Certain drugs such as nitrofurans are toxic to the heart muscle of baby birds, especially chukar and turkeys. Ascites is primarily seen in birds younger than 6 weeks.

Ascites can be induced in early brooding by faulty brooders (i.e., from lack of oxygen) or the rearing of gamebirds in high altitudes (low oxygen levels). As the heart muscle weakens, blood pressure decreases. The bird develops pulmonary congestion and abdominal ascites.

Mycotoxicosis of the liver and infectious hepatitis are known to result in ascites. Ascites in gamebirds is often associated with coliform omphalitis and cardiomyopathy in turkeys. Broiler chickens and meat-type ducklings appear genetically susceptible to the ascites because of the intense selection pressure for rapid growth.

CLINICAL SIGNS:

Early clinical signs are unthriftiness, lethargy, and weakness. At first, only an occasional bird will found dead, lying on its back. Mortality is greater between the ages of 2 to 5 weeks. The abdomen may be distended and feathers on the abdomen may be moist and soiled. Severely affected birds have difficulty breathing because of increased fluid in the lungs. The abdominal skin may be red; peripheral vessels congested; birds stunted, pulse and respiration rapid. Sudden death may occur before clinical signs are obvious.

PATHOLOGY:

Gross lesions include dilated flabby heart, fluid in the lungs, swollen liver, and gelatinous or ascitic fluid in the abdominal cavity. Lungs and liver are dark and congested. The edges of the liver are rounded. Lesions may be the result of increased fluid pressure on vital organs. The liver may be swollen and congested. Serum clots may adhere to the surface of the liver. There is pericarditis with adhesions in the pericardial (heart) sac.

If brooder pneumonia, microabscesses may be seen on cut surface of lung. The thymus and spleen are congested and the kidneys may be hemorrhagic. Birds that have died from ascites will have the characteristically enlarged heart, thickened right ventricle, fluid in the body cavities, and heart sac. Histologically, there is bile duct hyperplasia in the liver and aggregates of leukocytes in various tissues. Microscopic lesions are not diagnostic; but combined with history and gross lesions can confirm a diagnosis.

CONTROL:

Prevention of ascites requires the identification of the most-probable cause followed by appropriate corrective changes, whether management, infectious, or nutritional. If the cause is lack of oxygen, correct the brooding ventilation; if vitamin E-selenium deficiency, upgrade the feed; if an infectious process such as coliform omphalitis, focus on dirty eggs and incubator sanitation. Even heredity-induced ascites is helped by changing breeder pairings. When salt toxicity is found, check the water source and analyze the feed. DO NOT provide water treated with a water softener that uses salt for ion exchange to gamebirds and poultry. When hepatitis is the etiology, then one must determine whether it is an infection, mycotoxin, or drug toxicity.

DEHYDRATION

Dehydration is the pathophysiological response to a water deficit in the body. Many disease conditions result in excess loss of body water by fever, polyuria, vomiting, diarrhea, sweating, and hemorrhage. Any interference with water intake rapidly leads to signs of dehydration. The hotter the climate or room temperature, the shorter the time for onset of signs of dehydration and/or heat prostration.

The normal water consumption for birds is 2.5 times the feed intake. Birds will not eat when water is not available. Birds without feed will continue to drink, as water is essential to life. Water provides a great number of metabolic functions — aiding digestion, cooling the body, facilitating blood circulation, and providing catalytic action for enzymatic processes.

CLINICAL SIGNS:

Clinical signs of water deficiency are characteristic for all species of birds. Early signs of dehydration are doughy inelasticity of skin with dry mucous membranes. Other signs include a prolonged refill time for blood capillaries; the eyes become recessed into the sockets; and the extremities are cool. With 10 to 12 percent water loss, there is an exaggeration of these signs, as well as shock and muscle tremors. When water deficiency reaches 12 to 15 percent, acute shock and death occurs.

PATHOLOGY:

The diagnosis of dehydration is based on physical findings — weight loss, anorexia, elevated packed blood cell volume, and concentration of plasma protein. As dehydration continues, various metabolic functions become slow or stop and the affected bird or animal goes into renal failure, leading in turn to uremia and death. Histologically respective organ tissues are shrunken and exhibit congestion and blood cell concentration.

Many of the vital processes may be damaged beyond response to treatment. Oral administration is the preferred route; however, supplemental therapy can be injected parenterally (subcutaneously or by IV). Animals in shock should be given 5% dextrose solution. Plasma electrolytes should be monitored during IV rehydration.

CONTROL:

Dehydration can be controlled by providing adequate water and fountain space for all birds in each brood, flock, or pen. Be certain that there is a constant supply of fresh potable water for the birds. To encourage adequate water consumption, provide cool water in summer and protect water from freezing in winter.

Providing water to birds is a vital and important aspect of husbandry and management. Water is essential for normal growth, health, and immune response by gamebirds and poultry. The caretaker is responsible for supplying water as well as food, shelter, and protection for all captive birds on the farm.

DISSECTING ANEURYSM

A common fatal disease of semi-mature male turkeys and less frequently of gamebirds and chickens. The disease is characterized by internal hemorrhage as a result of the rupture of an aneurysm formed on the major vessels of healthy, thrifty birds. Death is sudden. Dissecting aneurysm may be called aortic rupture, **AR**, hypertension, or **DA**. The exact cause of rupture of an aortic aneurysm is unknown. Damage may be due to genetic hypertension (high blood pressure), copper deficiency, and/or toxic effects of beta aminopropionitrile (BAPN) and/or molybdenum (Mo) toxicity. Copper is essential for formation of connective tissue. BAPN occurs naturally in certain legumes, and is the only such plant substance known to contribute to the disease. High caloric and high-fat diets may contribute to or predispose birds to **DA**. Hypertension is a consistent finding in outbreak flocks with incidence in hypertensive lines about eight times that in hypotensive flocks. Birds must be fed to stimulate rapid growth which produces a prolonged lipemia that results in a rise in blood pressure. Aneurysm develops at the site of sclerotic plaques on inner walls of blood vessels. Susceptibility is concurrent with a period of rapid growth and early puberty; at this time, the impact of deficient nutrients, high blood fats, and/or toxic substances would be exaggerated. **DA** seems to be hereditary, as the incidence is higher in certain blood lines. The occurrence is worldwide wherever birds are grown and managed for maximum rate of gain. Outbreaks are sporadic and occur on a flock by flock basis. Nationally, the incidence is low. Dissecting aneurysm is not infectious, so there is no spread within the flock. The genetic predisposition (hypertension) is transmitted to progeny of breeder birds possessing these traits. Environmental and nutritional stresses may add to the severity of an outbreak.

CLINICAL SIGNS:

Death! Finding an apparently healthy bird dead is the first sign of trouble. Daily losses are low, but cumulative flock mortality may reach 10 percent. Occasionally a caretaker may observe a healthy bird that dies within minutes.

PATHOLOGY:

On necropsy, internal hemorrhage, bled-out tissue, and ruptured aorta are the primary findings. Gross lesions do not appear, as the birds were healthy until death. Aortic rupture usually occurs in the aorta between the external iliac and sciatic arteries. The damage is done when the aorta balloons or dilates at a spot that has lost strength and tone. Folds developing in the arterial lining partially obstruct the flow of blood, increasing pressure on the artery walls. Fatty arteriosclerotic-like substances are present in conjunction with folds in vessel lining. Diagnosis is based on flock history and confirmed by necropsy, massive blood clots in the abdominal cavity, and absence of other lesions. Adherent thrombi may be present at the site of the rupture. Rupture of smaller vessels are difficult to locate. Intimal thickening and fibrous plaques are present.

CONTROL:

Flock mortality can be reduced by lowering the energy intake and eliminating stress. Correct any mineral deficiencies, and add ascorbic acid to feed to enhance capillary integrity. Nutritional studies show that adding 200 ppm of copper to the diet will reduce incidence of **DA** in affected flocks. The combination of these measures will usually bring the condition under control. Select breeder replacements from known hypotensive breeds or lines. Review feed rations for breeders and young birds. Alter feeding program for birds between 16 to 23 weeks of age.

GOUT

Gout is an abnormal accumulation of urates in the tissues. Sodium urates are end products of protein digestion; they form in the kidneys and are eliminated in the feces. Gout occurs in two forms, articular and visceral.

Articular gout, generally restricted to individual birds, may be due to a genetic predisposition or a defect in uric acid metabolism. Some flock problems have been associated with very high protein levels in the diet.

Visceral gout occurs with renal failure after which all the urates are returned to the blood stream. A state of uremic poisoning exists and the urates are deposited on the surface of vital organs, especially the heart, liver, spleen, kidneys, and abdominal wall.

CLINICAL SIGNS:

Birds with articular gout have puffy joints, especially of the feet. The joints are enlarged and the feet appear abnormal. The bird usually does not exhibit pain in the affected joints or feet. Articular gout is common in older birds kept for pets. Visceral gout is usually discovered during necropsy.of dead birds. Some may have urate deposits in the vent area. These birds may have dry ruffled feathers and an unthrifty appearance.

PATHOLOGY:

Articular gout is characterized by deposits of urates around the joints. When incised, the periarticular tissues are white and the urate material is semi-fluid. Joint tissues are otherwise normal, and there are no typical arthritic lesions. Articular gout is associated with the feeding of a high-protein starter-type diet to adult and older birds that may have been kept for pets.

Visceral gout is characterized by white chalky deposits of urates on serosal surfaces, especially the heart, liver, and kidneys. This can be caused by kidney damage, blockage of ureters, or water deprivation. In commercial chickens, a nephrotoxic strain of infectious bronchitis plus simultaneous high-calcium feed causes the visceral gout; the condition is called urolithiasis Urinary calculi (stones) form in the ureters and block the flow of urine from the kidneys, causing pressure necrosis that destroys the kidneys. Shortly before death, uremic poisoning develops and urates are returned to the blood, then deposited on the organs. The lesions are found during necropsy of birds dead from urolithiasis.

CONTROL:

All gamebird producers should follow the nutritional recommendations for protein and calcium. Never provide more than 1 percent calcium to immature birds. Calcium in excess of 1 percent is needed only by breeder birds during production. Metabolically, birds need only the 1 percent calcium level for normal bone formation. Calcium in excess of that level becomes a stress and is excreted by the kidney. Any injury or kidney infection predisposes the bird to urolithiasis.

Likewise, protein in excess of that needed for growth and body maintenance is treated in the liver and converted to energy. The excess protein residues (sodium urates) are processed and excreted by the kidney.

Prolonged protein excess often produces articular gout. Vitamin **A** deficiency predisposes the kidney to gout problems. The best prevention against gout is a balanced diet for each stage of growth.

HEAT PROSTRATION

Any time a bird or animal is overcome by heat — from any source — the result is heat prostration or heat exhaustion. The cause could be heat from the sun or a enclosed environment with ventilation inadequate to control temperature and humidity, i.e., ventilation to expel the heat released by the birds.

Crowded gamebirds, meat-type young poultry, and birds in production are prime subjects to heat prostration, especially in the summer during periods of extreme heat. Birds have no sweat glands, and the only means of cooling is rapid respiration. If the body temperatures rise, the birds become weak and die from respiratory and circulatory failure or electrolyte imbalance. The normal body temperature of gamebirds and poultry is 105 to 107°F Fahrenheit.

Hot-day conditions make it difficult for birds to keep cool, and thus avoid being overcome by heat. When birds are overcome by heat, the brain's thermo-regulatory center that monitors body temperature fails to function, permitting body temperature to rise as high as 112°F. This creates a dangerous situation for the birds.

CLINICAL SIGNS:

Birds suffering from heat attempt to cool themselves by open-mouth breathing with wings relaxed loosely by the sides. Birds with heat prostration are weak and reluctant to move, but seek water and shade. Affected birds show shock, prostration, and death. Overcrowding during heat prostration results in high mortality. Mature, fat, and fleshy birds experience a high death rate. Daily mortality of as much as 25 percent has been reported.

PATHOLOGY:

Birds that die from heat prostration show multiple signs of tissue decomposition. The skeletal muscle will have wide whitish streaks (Zinker's necrosis). The heart, liver, spleen, kidneys, and brain will be swollen, congested, and hemorrhagic. The lungs are congested and the intestines will be flaccid and white with contents of a muco-catarrhal consistency. Birds with any form of illness at the time of heat stress are more susceptible to heat prostration. Body temperature may exceed the lethal 112°F.

CONTROL:

Preventive measures consist of adequate fans and ventilation ducts.

Every effort should be made to increase the air circulation. A combination of exhaust fans in the walls and in-line interior fans works well. The in-line fans provide air movement and exhaust fans remove the humidity exhaled by the birds. Air movement increased by 100 feet/second drops the air temperature by 1°, so increased air speed in the building will provide relief to the birds.

Other strategies for cooling the building are spraying the outside roof and walls, thus cooling the building by evaporation. Applying white or aluminum paint to the roof and outside walls also will help by reflecting the heat. For helpful cooling in commercial bird facilities, misting devices are used in conjunction with ventilation. Provide extra drinking fountains, and always avoid overcrowding.

IMPACTED GIZZARD

Impacted gizzard occurs when individual birds develop a depraved appetite and feed on nondigestible materials, e.g., litter, stones, or synthetic materials. Gizzard impaction can cause high mortality during the first 3 weeks in the lives of gamebirds, chicks, and poults. Hatchlings of different gamebird species tend to feed on the first materials they see when placed in the brooding pen. Affected birds become emaciated. The intestines are empty, but the gizzard will be a solid mass of fibrous materials. In most cases, impaction is confined to the gizzard.

CLINICAL SIGNS:

Litter-eating by baby birds is an early clinical sign of impaction. These birds become thin and emaciated, and die. On examination, they appear to have starved to death. Normal husbandry practice is to cover the litter under the brooding hover with paper or cloth and keep feed and water readily accessible, thus encouraging the hatchlings to eat the feed and ignore the litter. When hatchlings have learned to eat the feed rather than the litter, gizzard impaction rarely occurs. The primary signs are those associated with the starvation syndrome, i.e., emaciation, dehydration, ruffled feathers, weakness, and death.

PATHOLOGY:

Gross lesions are those of starvation — muscle atrophy, no food in digestive tract, and distended gall bladder. In young birds, the gizzard is impacted with litter, and in older birds, especially waterfowl, the gizzard will contain stones or other materials. There is an absence of infectious lesions. Microbiological cultures of blood and organs are negative for pathogenic organisms.

CONTROL:

Gizzard impaction is prevented by aggressive husbandry and management. The brooding facility must be cleaned and disinfected well in advance of the placement of baby gamebirds. The room should have clean bright new litter, chick guards in place around each hover, paper or cloth cover on the litter beneath the hovers, feeding and watering units filled and in place so as to be easily accessible to the baby birds — in other words, conditions as comfortable as possible for the birds under the hover. By the third or fourth day the birds should eating well and the covering material can be removed.

KERATOCONJUNCTIVITIS

Keratoconjunctivitis is the ulceration of the cornea (translucent part of eye), that commonly leads to blindness in gamebirds, ducklings, chickens, and turkeys. A synonym for keratoconjunctivitis is ammonia burn. The disease is caused by high levels of environmental ammonia produced by breakdown of the nitrogenous components of poultry manure. Ammonia levels of 50 ppm or greater are harmful to poultry. Along with causing keratoconjunctivitis, high ammonia levels damage the respiratory mucous membranes, increasing the flock's susceptibility to respiratory infections. High ammonia levels occur when management of litter and manure is neglected or ventilation in poultry housing is inadequate. When high ammonia levels persist, morbidity in gamebirds and chickens reaches 100 percent, turkeys 40 percent, and ducks 20 percent in the poultry house. Poultry of all ages are harmfully affected by high ammonia levels. Keratoconjunctivitis is a management disease of confined poultry that occurs wherever poultry is grown. There is no transmission of the disease since it is an in-house management (i.e., housekeeping) problem.

CLINICAL SIGNS:

Affected birds have difficulty moving because they have impaired vision. The eyes are continually watering (lachrymation). Facial swelling, edema of eyelids, corneal ulceration, and eventual blindness occur.

PATHOLOGY:

Lesions of Keratoconjunctivitis include ulceration of cornea of one or both eyes, inflammation of surrounding eye tissue (conjunctivitis), edema of eyelids, and mild tracheitis. Respiratory epithelial cells change from columnar to squamous, with loss of cilia. Partial to complete blindness occurs in advanced cases. A diagnosis is based on the history, clinical signs, and lesions, confirmed by measurements of ammonia levels in the poultry house. Twenty ppm is detectable to human smell.

CONTROL:

Keratoconjunctivitis can be controlled by replacing caked, wet litter with fresh, dry litter and increasing ventilation. Lesions will begin to regress when ammonia is removed. Vitamin A therapy will hasten repair of damage to the eyes and trachea. Spray litter or manure with a saponin compound to bind the ammonia.

Nitil, a natural tree resin saponin, can be safely administered in feed or water. It binds the nitrogen in feces, preventing ammonia release. With gamebirds, it is safe and effective from the first day to release or market.

Keratoconjunctivitis is prevented by husbandry that provides a healthful environment for gamebirds. This would include the use of Nitil liquid or other saponin plant products sprayed on litter and manure to prevent ammonia, more frequent removal of litter, and better ventilation.

MALABSORPTION

Malabsorption is a disease process, particularly of young birds, characterized by stunted growth and pale pigmentation of the skin. The condition has been diagnosed worldwide, but is more prevalent in areas where the bird population is highly concentrated.

Malabsorption is caused by a variety of etiological factors or agents. The viruses — including parvoviruses, astroviruses, calciviruses, rotaviruses, and/or reoviruses — are frequently involved. Mycotoxins and certain toxic plant substances are also causes. The reoviruses and mycotoxins are the most commonly diagnosed causes. Reoviruses are prevalent throughout the world with the manifestation in other disease forms, such as helicopter disease of chicks and poults, viral septicemia in caged layers, and ruptured tendon syndrome in roaster chickens.

The reoviruses tend to be species specific. The chicken group shares a common group antigen that is useful in recognition and diagnosis. Transmission occurs by oral and respiratory routes as well as vertically from infected breeder hens. The virus increases virulence within the flock.

Mycotoxins produce malabsorption and paleness by interfering with digestion and nutrient absorption, as well as increasing capillary fragility, hemorrhage, and anemia. Fusarium-origin T-2 mycotoxin causes a severe problem in young gamebirds and poultry.

CLINICAL SIGNS:

Malabsorption syndrome is typically recognized in young gamebirds and poultry between 1 and 6 weeks of age. The disease is characterized by a slower or stunted growth pattern; and also causes osteoporosis and poor digestion.

Affected birds develop pale, nonpigmented skin coloring, feather abnormalities (helicopter disease), undigested (unabsorbed) feed in the feces, stiff gait, arthritis, tenosynovitis, osteoporosis, and diarrhea. Diarrhea is usually one of the first signs; evidenced by feed passing undigested. Mortality rates for the flock increase as well as a general unevenness in sizes of the birds within the flock. Severely affected birds may not respond to feed changes or management practices. Flock appearance can be improved by culling and removing severely stunted and sick birds. These birds can be submitted to the diagnostic laboratory for clinical diagnosis.

PATHOLOGY:

Lesions from viral infections are more pronounced in the intestines where cytopathic effect can be observed histologically on the mucosal lining of the gut. There is a loss of villi, an increase of goblet (i.e., mucin) cells, and an invasion of the wall with edema, erythrocytes, and heterophils. Other clinical signs develop as a result of the damage in the intestine that reduces digestion, absorption, and utilization of nutrients. Direct action by the virus also produces hepatitis, pancreatitis, myocarditis, arthritis, osteoporosis, and necrosis of the intestinal villi. Atrophy of the gizzard and proventriculus are common in older recovered birds. Encephalomalacia has been reported subsequent to malabsorption when Vitamin E fails to be absorbed.

A presumptive diagnosis can be based on farm and flock history, clinical signs, and gross lesions. More conclusive evidence requires the isolation and identification of the virus or other causal agent. Virus can be propagated in the yolk sacs of 5- to 7-day-old chicken embryos or demonstrating the virus in the feces from the on histopathological examination of the diarrheic birds by electron microscopy (EM). Other diagnostic laboratory procedures should be used as developed by the respective laboratory.

CONTROL:

Severely affected birds may not respond to changes in feed and/or management practices. Flock appearance improves by culling and removing the severely stunted and sick birds. Such birds can be submitted to the diagnostic laboratory for clinical diagnosis. Control requires:

Treating flock treatment by dietary supplementation with water-dispersible fat- and water-soluble vitamins. Antibiotics are recommended for intestinal infections.

Providing new feed, from a new supplier.

Managing litter to eliminate wet spots.

Ensure maximum comfort for the birds through practice of good husbandry

MYOPATHIES

Myopathies are degenerative changes and replacement of muscle tissue by fat and connective (scar) tissue. Gamebirds and poultry present a variety of myopathy problems. Myopathy conditions are more prevalent and severe in domestic species of birds genetically selected for rapid growth and fed diets that provide maximum rates of growth.

Some environments for birds are designed to require minimal energy for body-heat production, permitting a total focus on growth rate with minimal exercise or physical exertion expected of the bird. Several bird myopathies, caused by a deficiency of vitamin E and selenium in the diet, are called 'White Muscle Disease.' Vitamin E and selenium function as antioxidants that protect the cell membrane from damage by 'peroxides' that form from digestive action.

CLINICAL SIGNS:

Clinical signs vary according to the form of myopathy, cause, and with the organ or skeletal structure affected.

WHITE MUSCLE DISEASE (WMD): Damage from WMD is reflected in the degeneration of the heart, gizzard, and skeletal muscles. The heart becomes rounded and bulbous. Gizzard muscle becomes pale with a degeneration of muscle bundles. Skeletal muscle becomes pale with whitish streaks throughout.

WMD is a deficiency disorder; in baby chickens, the amino acid cystiene has been implicated. Cardiomyopathy (i.e., flabby heart syndrome) is suspected with subcutaneous edema of lower abdomen, ascites, and sudden death of healthy thrifty birds. Broilers and turkeys have a higher-than-average incidence of myopathies; thus, confirming a genetic component for the disorder.

TOXIC MYOPATHY: Clinical signs of toxic myopathy are lameness, leg deformities, crippling, abnormal skeletal development, hock-joint abnormalities, weakness, depression, stunting and paresis. Ionophere (monensin) toxicity causes muscle damage with depression, weakness, and an inability of the bird to rise. Birds become paretic (paralyzed) as the condition progresses. Respiratory distress occurs when muscles of inhalation are affected.

DEEP PECTORAL MYOPATHY: Lack of physical exercise contributes to deep pectoral myopathy (green muscle disease) in commercial strains of turkeys. Flock incidence of 25 percent has been reported in turkeys of market age. As heavy birds run, jump, and attempt to fly, they rupture the deep pectoral muscle, causing hemorrhage, swelling, and edema. The defect can be identified by a depression (dimpling) of the breast over the affected muscle, noticed at slaughter.

RUPTURED TENDON (RT): RT, also called viral arthritis, occurs primarily in heavy birds that are down because of lameness or leg deformity. Grossly, the leg muscles are firm and pale. The condition is referred to as GREEN LEG SYNDROME, since the leg turns green during the healing process. The tendon of the gastrocnemius leg muscle atrophies and pulls away from the attachment to the muscle that causes the hemorrhage at the time of rupture. Bilateral rupture is frequent.

PATHOLOGY:

WHITE MUSCLE DISEASE: On post-mortem examination, the heart is grossly enlarged, rounded, thin-walled, and flabby. Microscopic changes include swelling, edema, hyalinization, mineralization, and degeneration of the muscle fibers, plus infiltration of white blood cells into the lesion. Hypercellularity from sarcolemmal nuclei may be prominent if regeneration is occurring.

TOXIC MYOPATHY: Most of the skeletal muscles, neck, legs, and tail, are affected. Lesions may be found in the heart muscles. Gross and histological muscle changes are similar to those of WMD. Histologically affected muscles show degeneration with fragmentation of the myofibrils.

DEEP PECTORAL MYOPATHY: Rupture of deep pectoral muscles during growth results in hemorrhage, swelling, edema, followed with degeneration of the muscle fibers. The muscle turns green from resorption of the hemorrhaged blood. The condition is found when the bird is slaughtered and is identified by a depression over the site of the damaged muscle. Histologically, the damaged muscle becomes encapsulated resulting in dry, green, necrotic muscles enclosed in a thick fibrous capsule.

RUPTURED TENDON: The hemorrhage is purplish, then turns green as blood components are resolved. The ruptured tendon can be palpated as a hard mass on the back of the leg above the hock. Histological finds are swelling, hyalinization, muscle fiber and tendon necrosis, and edema. As the lesions progress, heterophils and macrophage WBCs move into the lesions. Virus can be isolated from the diseased tendon. Affected birds are seropositive for reovirus.

CONTROL:

Myopathies require that the primary condition be identified as to probable etiology. Then a specific treatment, based on the respective cause, can follow.

WMD control requires a correction of the diet of the affected flock as well as a correction of the ration for the breeder flock. Specific medication is dietary supplementation of Vitamin E in the water and followed with addition of vitamin E and selenium to the feed. Seriously affected birds do not recover but proper treatment stops the development of new cases. The rule of thumb is when five birds per thousand are affected, the ration should be checked. The rule applies for any trace element deficiency. Treatment is recommended for commercial flocks and for individual birds in a hobby flock.

TOXIC MYOPATHY: Control requires the discovery and removal of the toxic material. Ionophore toxicity occurs when the feed is not properly mixed (hot spots), use of excessive levels of the compound, and/or miscalculation of the dosage. Slaughter recovered gamebirds.

Change to new nonmedicted feed. Because the drug settles to the bottom, be sure to empty and clean all feed troughs. To avoid development of new cases, provide a vitamin-pack treatment in the water. Sulfa toxicity requires the removal of sulfa drugs and provision of fresh clean water for 2 days. Then administer vitamins for 2 days to detoxify birds. Same procedure is recommended for any toxic substance. T-2 mycotoxins require the replacement of feed with fresh feed that is mycotoxin-free. Do not administer antibiotics. Salt poisoning requires the removal of the source of salt. If feed is the source, change feed. If water is the source, find a new source of water. Water from many farm wells are high in salt. Normally, 0.5 percent salt is the recommendation for gamebirds.

DEEP PECTORAL MYOPATHY: Provide additional space per bird in flocks confined in buildings. Administer supplemental vitamin-electrolytes and hematinic substances to replace lost blood cells.

RUPTURED TENDON: To control reovirus, immunize breeder flocks and vaccinate all heavy meat (roaster) flocks scheduled for market; practice all-in, all-out production program; and thorough C&D after terminating the RT flock. Dietary vitamin-electrolyte supplements are recommended. Antibiotics are optional, if used at half-dose level. Remove crippled birds.

NONSPECIFIC ENTERITIS

Enteritis, inflammation of the intestines, is not a specific disease. It is part of the clinical syndrome of many diseases. "Enteritis unidentified" is a synonym.

A wide variety of agents causes enteritis, and in those cases where a known pathogen is found, the disease is diagnosed as such. Diseases that commonly cause enteritis as part of the clinical picture are coccidiosis; intestinal parasitism; histomoniasis; trichomoniasis; hexamitiasis; various fungi; various bacteria including paratyphoid, *Salmonella arizona*, coliforms, and anaerobes. Transmissible and hemorrhagic enteritis of turkeys are examples of an enteric virus.

The term "nonspecific enteritis" is used to denote the condition when the cause cannot be identified. Poultry of all ages are susceptible, but the disease is more common in birds older than 12 weeks, especially those kept in unsanitary pens and/or infected with other unrecognized intestinal disorders. Enteritis occurs worldwide, wherever poultry are grown. The mode of transmission is specific to the disease agent.

CLINICAL SIGNS:

General unthriftiness as denoted by dirty ruffled feathers, paleness, diarrhea, poor growth or egg production, drop in feed and water consumption, and a slight increase in daily flock mortality.

PATHOLOGY:

The pathological changes are confined to the digestive tract. Typical lesions include hemorrhage, tumors, adhesions, peritonitis, intestinal walls that are thickened, inflamed, and flaccid, necrosis or ulceration of the mucosa, and intestinal contents that are catarrhal, fetid, and caseous. Various sections of intestine may be affected: duodenum, jejunum, ileum, ceca, colon, and cloaca. The diagnosis is based on symptoms and typical lesions as well as other intestinal lesions. If the cause is unknown, and intestinal lesions are found, the condition is diagnosed as "nonspecific enteritis" and is thought to be caused by ingestion of high numbers of filth organisms. Organisms prevalent in filth are usually found in routine culturing and isolation procedures involving the disease.

CONTROL:

Short-term medication and practice of good hygiene help to control enteritis. When enteritis breaks, identification of the specific cause should be made, if possible. The drug selected, such as neomycin, must work against a wide range of organisms, yet provide a wide safety margin and not be readily absorbed into the bloodstream. In addition to neomycin, the list of drugs frequently prescribed includes tetracycline, bacitracin, penicillin, sulfa drugs, and in certain cases, water sanitizers. Supportive medication with vitamins and electrolytes also speeds recovery of the flock.

Start medication without delay, prevent stress, upgrade hygiene, and environment. Prevention is best achieved by excellent husbandry with special attention to good hygiene, litter management, potable water, fresh feed, and proper ventilation.

PHOTOSENSITIZATION

Photosensitization is a condition in which lightly pigmented skin becomes hyperactive to sunlight due to a photodynamic agent in the skin. Molecules of photosensitizing agents are energized by light, transfering the energy to receptor molecules and initiating a chemical reaction in the skin cells.

Photosensitivity is not the same as sunburn. With sunburn, the skin cells become inflamed by the ultraviolet rays. While photosensitization is not a common in gamebirds, the disease does occur worldwide in poultry. It is important to the gamebird industry in that many bird dogs are quite susceptible to photosensitization.

CLINICAL SIGNS: Photosensitive animals are photophobic when exposed to sunlight. The animal's skin blisters and forms scabs, and then becomes necrotic. Mammals can develop glossitis (inflamation of the tongue) from licking the blistered skin. If the photosensitivity is related to the animal's diet, the liver may be damaged (toxic) and an icterus (jaundice) will develop.

PATHOLOGY: Blisters and necrosis of the skin are the primary lesions. Most lesions are confined to the lightly pigmented areas of the skin. Mammals, especially dogs and sheep, are the primary animals affected. In these cases, eyelids, nose (muzzle), ears, and white skin areas are severely affected. Sunlight exposure is always involved regardless of the sensitizing agent. Certain inbred lines may be more sensitive than other breeds or species.

CONTROL: Initial treatment is to shield the affected animal from sunlight. Examine the ration for drugs or additives known to sensitize animals to sunlight. The skin lesions should heal quite well, even after extensive necrosis. The prognosis and eventual productivity of an animal are related to the severity of the lesions and the quality of the healing. Since hunting dogs are susceptible, gamebird growers and hunting preserve operators must be alert for the condition.

When in doubt, check it out. Veterinarians will readily recognize photosensitization and can prescribe specific treatment.

REPRODUCTIVE DISORDERS

The following are reproductive disorders associated with gamebird production.

ABNORMAL EGGS

SOFT-SHELLED or SHELL-LESS EGGS are caused by T-2 mycotoxicosis, blood poisoning, calcium deficiency, or acute infections such as avian influenza.

DOUBLE-YOLKED EGGS are caused by malfunction of the ovary timing. (Normally, the ovary releases a single yolk at 26-hour intervals.) Occasionally a hen lays double-yolked eggs during the same clutch. Usually, only a few hens in the flock produce these eggs.

EGGS WITH TWO OR MORE SHELLS. The cause is not known. Wrinkled shell, calcium deposit on the shell, and egg containing a worm. (Occasionally an intestinal worm will move up the oviduct and become trapped in an egg as it is formed. This is not a disease. It is a chance occurrence, detectable when candled.) The wrinkled shell is an after-effect of IB or magnesium imbalance in the diet. The mineral deposits may result from ingesting excessive calcium, such as 4% calcium in the feed.

BLOOD OR MEAT SPOTS IN EGG. Blood clots result from follicle hemorrhage at the time of ovulation. Meat spots are a result of bits of the oviduct mucosa. Blood occurs on the yolk and meat spots in the albumin.

IMPACTED OVIDUCT (EGG BOUND)

Caused by paralysis of the oviduct muscles, or by partial twisting (torsion) of the oviduct. Unlaid eggs become lodged in the oviduct, or the oviduct becomes atonic and unable to expel eggs. Eggs accumulate, causing gross distention of the oviduct and abdomen of the hen. Upon necropsy, the oviduct is found to be filled with semi-dry egg concretions (fluid part of the egg is reabsorbed, leaving the solid components to compact the oviduct).

INTERNAL LAYERS

Usually a result of yolk falling into the abdominal cavity of the hen when it is forced from the funnel portion (infundibulum) of the oviduct. Occurrence is rather common in high producing and/or flighty hens. Occasional occurrence will not cause death of the hen, but chronic internal layers die from peritonitis.

EGG YOLK PERITONITIS

Causes death of laying hens. The egg yolk ruptures before entering the oviduct, spilling yolk material over the viscera. Peritonitis develops and causes death. Occurrence is sporadic. The condition is associated with certain septicemic diseases, including reovirus septicemia, fowl cholera, staphylococcosis, and rough handling of excitable breeders after onset of production.

EVERSION (PROLAPSE) OF THE OVIDUCT

Prolapsed oviduct, blowout, or pick-out problems are most common in pullets and young hens. Prolapsed oviduct results from straining during and/or following the laying process. Prolapse is caused by:

LARGE EGGS LAID BY SMALL HENS. Occurs most frequently with prolonged delay of sexual maturity in pullets. They start their lay with large eggs; invariably, there is high incidence of prolapse.

EXTREME OBESITY. Fat in the pelvis and lower abdomen produces partial obstruction of the production pathway, causing strain.

AFTER EFFECT OF IMPACTION. Swelling and irritation of the oviduct that causes the hen to continue to strain after the egg is laid.

VENT PICKING. Most common cause of oviduct prolapses in high-production flocks. No beak trim or improper beak trim leads to cannibalism and high incidence of prolapses. Flocks maintained on the floor, mismanagement practices that lead to cannibalism include insufficient nest space and poor positioning of the nest bar. Hens standing on the nest bar should not be able to pick at hens that are on the nest.

ENTERITIS AND CLOACITIS. Chronic irritation of the cloaca will cause straining that leads to prolapsing. Vent gleet (candidiasis, a yeast infection of the vent) is a common infection of the cloacal area.

TUMORS OF THE LOWER ABDOMINAL REGION are common in flocks infected with leukosis.

HEREDITARY PREDISPOSITION. Very rare.

ACCELERATED LIGHTING PROGRAM in young hens.

SALPINGITIS

Inflammation of the oviduct, characterized by a foul-smelling exudate in the vent region. Caused by a variety of infectious agents. Bacteria from the intestinal tract, including salmonellae, are common causes. In young growing pullets, salpingitis often follows outbreaks of *Mycoplasma gallisepticum*. Lesions at necropsy include peritonitis, metritis (inflammation of the uterus), and oviduct filled with a whitish-yellow thick, tenacious exudate. In chronic cases, exudate (pus) may be caseous or dry.

OOPHORITIS

Inflammation of the ovary is associated with pullorum disease and fowl typhoid. Characterized by irregularly shaped, shrunken, greenish-discolored ova.

CYSTIC RIGHT OVIDUCT

Common after-effect of infectious bronchitis. In the avian female, the right oviduct is only a vestigial (undeveloped) organ, containing a minute amount of clear sterile fluid. Following IB outbreaks, the right oviduct may become quite large and accumulate up to 1 to 3 ounces of a clear to milky-colored fluid and whitish-yellow solids.

ROUND HEART DISEASE

Round Heart Disease (RHD) is a spontaneous cardiomyopathy of young birds, especially turkeys and chickens. The disease is characterized by cardiac arrest and sudden death. The exact cause is unknown, but factors that contribute include genetic predisposition, hypoxia during incubation and brooding, and nitrofuran toxicity in new hatchlings. Other implicated, but not confirmed, causes are hereditary trypsin inhibition, and viral myocarditis. High altitude readily causes RHD in fast growing broiler chickens in which hypoxia is considered to be the underlying cause.

CLINICAL SIGNS:

The first sign of RHD may be may be sudden death. Most deaths occur during the first 4 weeks after hatching. Although death from RHD is sudden, some birds may show ruffled feathers, droopy wings, lethargy, labored breathing, and gasping just before dying. As birds become older, deaths are more sporadic. Overall, the brood of young birds appears thrifty and healthy. Individual birds with the defective heart are the only birds affected.

PATHOLOGY:

The lesions of RHD are found when dead birds are necropsied. Characteristically, the affected bird will have a grossly enlarged and rounded heart. The lungs will be congested and the liver swollen. Other findings may include ascites (fluid in abdomen), generalized edema, pulmonary edema, and hydro-pericardium. All lesions are caused by the weakened heart action and a drop in blood pressure.

In older birds, the enlarged heart may be the sole and primary lesion. Histologically, general myopathy of the heart is nonspecific. Heart changes include muscle degeneration, congestion, and lymphoid infiltrates. Diagnosis is based on history, gross lesions, and absence of other disease or conditions.

CONTROL:

There is no specific treatment for RHD. Have feed analysed to assure adequate Vitamin E, selenium, and sodium. Check for presence of nitrofurazone and/or polychlorinated biphenyl. Provide recommended husbandry and hygiene procedures. Give soluble vitamins and electrolytes in the drinking water for 2 to 5 days. Initiate other antistress procedures. Keep room temperature at comfortable level for the birds.

GROWER'S REFERENCE

ON

GAMEBIRD HEALTH

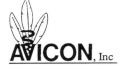

AVICON, Inc

POISONOUS AND TOXIC SUBSTANCES

OVERVIEW

Poisonous and toxic substances have been recognized for hundreds of years. Toxicology is the study of the effects of poisons on animals and plants. The TOXIC AGENT, or TOXICANT, causes an illness called toxicosis in animals or humans that inhale or swallow it. Some powerful toxins produced by plants (e.g., poison oaks and ivies) cause harm if they touch the skin. The term TOXIN is used for poisonous compounds produced by a biological source such as venom, plant toxins, or botulism toxin.

If the word HAZARD appears on the label, it implies the likelihood of poisoning in current conditions of the use of the substance. The current concept is that it is the size of the DOSE that makes the poison. This is an easy concept with known toxic materials but it is also true with products used to stimulate growth such as chemicals and chemotherapeutic agents considered safe for use as growth stimulants.

A toxic overdose will cause illness. A misplaced decimal in the calculation for medication in water or feed, e.g., can cause toxicosis. Inversely, the medication may be so slight that it has no effect on the disease.

Drugs, minerals, vitamins, heavy metals, and pesticides are often involved in food poisoning, allergic reactions, or photosensitization. It has long been known that salt (NaCL) and the vitamins **A** and **D** are safe for use in moderate amounts, but are frequently toxic in high doses. Many of the trace elements (feed nutrients such as selenium, for example) needed for optimum growth are toxic in higher doses.

Poisonous substances are widely distributed in nature. Mycotoxins are emerging as important and common toxicants. Poisoning occurs more frequently in birds on free-range and in backyard flocks in villages where birds forage on neighborhood gardens and garbage-disposal sites.

This section covers antibiotics, drugs, heavy metals, mycotoxins, pesticides, and rodenticides. Botulism, even though a toxin, is caused by a bacterium, and is covered in the section on bacterial diseases.

MOLDS (FUNGI)

Mycologists (scientists who study fungi) have identified more than 80,000 kinds of molds. Fungi are found in all parts of the world. Some are beneficial and some are harmful, depending on the species and conditions of growing. Although classed as plants, molds do not have the chlorophyll that gives leaf tissues in higher plants their green color, and enables them to convert the energy of sunlight into plant food. Because molds cannot manufacture their food, they must live where they can feed on nutrients already present. Although usually found on dead or decayed plant and animal material, some molds live as parasites on and in living plants and animals. It is in this role that they can cause diseases in gamebirds.

With favorable temperature and moisture levels, molds can live on practically all types of materials. Metals and plastics are the only substances known to be free of attack by molds.

Molds play leading roles in the decay of dead plants and animals, converting the dead tissues into nutrients for other plants and organisms.

Most mold species reproduce by forming spores. Most of these are extremely prolific spore-formers and can reproduce at much faster rates than most of the higher plants and animals. Spores are microscopic and ideally configured for riding air currents. Living spores have been trapped more than 7 miles above the earth's surface. Wind movement is the primary method by which mold spores move to new locations, incubate, grow, and make new spores.

In general, molds are well adapted to living at various temperatures, but sensitive to high temperatures. Exposure to temperatures ranging between 160 and 212°F will destroy most molds. On the other hand, low temperatures do not kill molds. Most will stop growing at temperatures cooler than 40°F, but do not die. When the temperature becomes warm, they resume growth and reproduction. Molds require a certain amount of moisture, but they can grow on seeds, flour, wood, leather, and a host of other materials of very low moisture content if the relative humidity of the air is 70 percent or higher. Controlling humidity is one important method of avoiding trouble with molds. Knowledge regarding the role of molds in many poultry diseases is far from complete, but research in this area is continuing in the effort to expand understanding and effectiveness of control.

Molds that are pathogenic or produce toxins harmful to gamebirds and poultry include: Aspergillus and Candida (see under "Bacterial and Fungal Diseases," p 33, and "Mycotoxins," below).

MYCOTOXINS

Mycotoxicosis is a serious condition in gamebirds and poultry of any age. It is the result of ingesting mycotoxins, a poisonous substance produced on feedstuffs by certain molds. The toxic effect is cumulative, and the malady is characterized by vague symptoms and non-specific lesions.

Mycotoxins are toxins produced by pathogenic fungi. Illness results from ingestion of the toxin, not from eating the mold itself. Molds are found everywhere. More than 100 different mycotoxins have been identified; but only three groups of mycotoxins [aflatoxins, ochratoxins, and fusariotoxins] are predominantly involved in gamebird health problems. Molds readily grow on most feed ingredients. Incidence and rate of growth are dependent on moisture, temperature, and nature of the substrate (i.e., the feedstuff). Most molds grow in temperatures of from 40° to 120°F, if relative humidity is at least 75 percent. When humidity is less than 65 percent, growth is inhibited.

Specific information about mycotoxins that affect gamebirds:

AFLATOXINS — Several different aflatoxins are produced by mold strains of *Aspergillus flavus* and *A. parasiticus*. B_1, B_2, G_1, and G_2 are the more common types. B_1 is the most common, as well as the most toxic. It is a problem in migratory waterfowl, especially when feeding in peanut harvest fields.

OCHRATOXIN — Produced by *Aspergillus ochraceus* and *Penicillium viridicatium*. Growth requirements of the mold and the effects of its toxin on birds parallel those of aflatoxin. Only one toxin has been identified in ochratoxicosis, Ochratoxin **A**. It is characterized as a nephrotoxin.

FUSARIOTOXINS — Fusarium molds are the most common infective molds of grains during cool, wet weather. The fusariotoxins that affect gamebirds are:

ZEARALENONE — This toxin, also known as **F-2**, is produced by *Fusarium roseum* and is estrogenic in that it can lead to reproductive disorders.

T-2 TOXIN — Trichothecene-type compounds are skin irritants that cause mouth lesions and reproductive failures.

SCIRPENOLS — Another group of trichothecene-type of

compounds.

FURASINS — Toxic compounds produced by*Fusarium monoliforme.*

FUMONISINS — Compounds produced by strains of*F. monoliforme.*

Poultry of all ages, gamebirds, waterfowl, animals, and humans are susceptible but the degree of susceptibility varies from species to species. Newly hatched and very young gamebirds are extremely susceptible to aflatoxins and ochratoxins, while older poultry are seriously affected by T-2 toxins. Mycotoxins damage the immune system causing birds to be more susceptible to infections. Transmission is by ingesting mycotoxins.

CLINICAL SIGNS:

Vary from unthriftiness, paleness of shanks and combs, to paralysis.

AFLATOXICOSIS in young birds retards growth and causes anemia (paleness). Depressed growth and reductions in feed efficiency will appear within 17 days. Capillaries become fragile, resulting in hemorrhage, bruising, and regressing of the bursa of Fabricius. Production and fertility drop in breeder birds.

OCHRATOXICOSIS produces stunting, anemia, and capillary fragility. Concentrations as low as 1 ppm cause bruising in broilers, similar to aflatoxicosis. Toxin at a level of 4 ppm depresses growth rate and increases mortality in young birds.

FUSARIUM T-2 MYCOTOXIN is an irritant and inflammatory agent. Canker-type lesions at the commissures (corners) of the mouth and scabby lesions on feet and shanks may be the first clinical signs.

SCIRPENOLS depress growth, egg production, and increase mortality.

FUSARINS (particularly Fusarin C) are mutagenic, cause heart and liver lesions, and death.

FUMONISINS B_1 is considered to be the causative agent of equine leucoencephalomalacia. Twenty ppm of dietary fumonisin causes mortality in young birds.

PATHOLOGY:

AFLATOXIN in day-old ducklings produces hepatic (liver) tumors. Other lesions are hepatomas, anemia (pale bone marrow), muscle weakness, capillary fragility, enteritis, hemorrhagic syndrome, and encephalitis.

OCHRATOXICOSIS produces the anemia-hemorrhage-bruising effect described for aflatoxicosis. Weights of the internal organs increase. The toxin is confirmed by chemical assay.

FUSARIUM T-2 mycotoxin is not detectable by ultraviolet light. Mold is visible on the tips of diseased ears of corn.

CONTROL:

Effective treatment depends on removal of the source of mycotoxin, i.e., removal of the contaminated feed. Flock improvement will follow. Adding mold inhibitors is helpful. Administration of water-dispersible, fat-soluble vitamins A, D, E, and K is recommended. Mycotoxins, especially T-2, prevent absorption of these fat-soluble vitamins from the feed. Watching for signs of mycotoxicosis and an on-going feed-monitoring program are the best preventive actions. There is an essential link between food quality and health in any animal.

FOLLOWING ARE GUIDELINES FOR FEED HANDLING:

Use mold inhibitors in the feed.

Store feed ingredients in clean, dry facilities.

If bin temperatures build up, immediately begin aeration (i.e., cooling).

Keep all equipment for mixing, transporting, and storing feed clean. This will prevent buildup of caked moldy feed. Use a disinfectant such as 10% Clorox solution or propionate solution [2 oz/gal].

Adjust automatic feeders so that the amount of feed delivered to the birds is adequate but not in excess. Force the birds to clean up the feed each day.

-- IMPORTANT --

Feedstuffs contaminated with mycotoxins cannot be "fixed." Cooking or heating contaminated feedstuffs will destroy the mold organisms, but the toxins remain. In general, feedstuffs contaminated with mycotoxins are dangerous for other animals. Dispose of toxin-contaminated feed in the same manner as spent litter.

DRUGS (OVERDOSE)

Drugs are manufactured medicinals. They do not occur in nature. Drugs are chemically synthesized and manufactured by pharmaceutical companies, then marketed for use in treatment and control of specific infectious diseases of gamebirds, poultry, livestock, and humans. Drugs constitute the majority of all medicines available for treatment and control of diseases. Even though drugs seemingly can perform miracles, the spectrum of activity is limited. Specific drugs are designed for specific uses.

The following listing enumerates effective DRUGS; the diseases or syndromes in which the drug is effective called ACTIVITY; the side effects if the drug is improperly used as TOXICITY; and the amount of the drug with method of administration as DOSAGE.

SULFA DRUGS

ACTIVITY: Coccidia, Salmonella, Pasteurella, and Coliform bacteria

TOXICITY: Depression, paleness, aplastic anemia, pale bone marrow, nephrosis (crystals forming in kidneys), egg-shell depigmentation, and death.

DOSAGE: GAMEBIRDS AND TURKEYS: 57 g/ton (.00625%) in feed.

CHICKENS: 113.5 g/ton (0.0125%) in feed.

DUCKS: 227 - 454 g/ton (0.025 - 0.05%) in feed

Sulfadimethoxine (Albon) 12.5 % Liquid

GAMEBIRDS AND TURKEYS: 1 oz/4 gal in water for 5 days

CHICKENS: 1 oz/2 gal in water for 5 days

DUCKS: 1 oz/1 gal in water for 5 days

Other Sulfas (SQ, Sulmet)

Same dose — BUT with an intermittent schedule — 3 DAYS ON/2 DAYS OFF, 2 DAYS ON/2 DAYS OFF etc. for 7 days' TOTAL MEDICATION.

NITROFURANS

**FURAZOLIDONE,
NITROFURAZONE (NF-180, NFZ)**

ACTIVITY: Clostridia, Salmonella, Coliform, Staphyloccocus,
             Streptococcus

TOXICITY: Depression, growth retardation, nervous signs,
             ataxia, heart damage (round heart), death

DOSAGE: 50 - 200 g/ton for 5 to 7 days in feed
             100 mg/gal for 5 to 7 days in water
             (Dilute according to guide on label)

NOTE: Repeat later if needed

COCCIDIOSTATS

**AMPROLIUM
(AMPROL, CORID)**

ACTIVITY: Most species of coccidia

TOXICITY: Hyperexcitability, neurological signs (head over back)
             Interferes with Thiamine (Vitamin B_1) utilization. Signs
             reversible — withdraw amprol or medicate with
             vitamins in drinking water.

DOSAGE: PHEASANTS: (120 g/ton) (0.0175% level) in feed.

             CHICKENS AND TURKEYS: (117-234 g/ton) (0.125%-
             0.025% level) in feed.

             NOTE: Follow dilution instructions on product label if
                   administering these coccidiostats in water.

**CLOPIDOL
(COYDEN-25, METICLOPINDOL)**

ACTIVITY: All species of coccidia, Avian Malaria

TOXICITY: Coccidia resistance — loss of effectiveness

DOSAGE: CHICKENS: 0.0125%-0.025% level in feed.

             NOTE: This material not available for administration in
             water.

HALOFUGINONE
(STENOROL)

ACTIVITY: All species of coccidia, Avian Malaria

TOXICITY: Depression, nervousness, unthriftiness

DOSAGE: CHICKENS: 0.0003% level; 2.72 g/ton in feed

TURKEYS: 0.00015%- 0.0003% level; 1.36-2.72 g/ton in feed

NOTE: Halofuginone is not available for administration in water.

NOTE: This material is not cleared for gamebirds

IONOPHORES:
(COBAN, SALINOMYCIN, LASALOCID,
NARASIN, MANDURAMICIN)

ACTIVITY: Coccidiostats; All species of coccidia/ antibacterial

TOXICITY: Depression, weakness, paresis, sternal recumbancy with legs extended backwards, severe damage to heart, leg muscles, toxic myopathy, and dyspnea in turkeys. Toxicity focus is damage to muscle. Lethal to horses.

DOSAGE: QUAIL: Coban [73 g/ton] in feed for 10 weeks

NOTE: COBAN IS CLEARED
ONLY FOR USE WITH QUAIL

CHICKENS: 90 - 110 g/ton in feed for 8 weeks

TURKEYS: 54 - 90 g/ton in feed for 10 weeks

NOTE: This material not available for administration in water. At this time, ionophores have limited FDA clearance for use in gamebirds

ARSENICAL FEED ADDITIVES (OVERDOSE)

NOTE: ARSENICAL COMPOUNDS ARE LETHAL TO WATERFOWL, PIGEONS, AND DOGS.

PHENYLARSONIC ACID:

ARSANILIC ACID, ROXARSONE, CARBARSONE, CARBOSEP, HISTOSTAT

NOTE: THESE MATERIALS ARE NEITHER CLEARED NOR RECOMMENDED FOR GAMEBIRDS.

ACTIVITY: Growth, prevention of histomoniasis

TOXICITY: Clinical signs induced by an overdose or lack of water during medication, especially in hot weather, are neuropathy, lameness, weakness, staggering, and incoordination.

DOSAGE: CHICKENS and TURKEYS: 22.7 - 45.4 g/ton in feed.

NOTE: THESE MATERIALS ARE NOT USED IN DRINKING WATER.

NICARBAZIN AND ZOALENE

NOTE: NICARBAZIN AND ZOALENE ARE NOT RECOMMENDED FOR GAMEBIRDS.

ACTIVITY: Coccidiostat

TOXICITY: Listless, dull, ataxic, anorexia. In adult birds, egg production drops, shell pigments are lost, hatchability is reduced, and yolks mottle.

DOSAGE: CHICKENS: 0.0125% level in feed
TURKEYS: 0.01875% level in feed

NOTE: THESE MATERIALS ARE NOT USED IN DRINKING WATER.

DIMETRIDAZOLE
EMTRYL, NITRAZOLE

NOTE: THIS MATERIAL IS NOT AVAILABLE IN THE USA.

ACTIVITY: Control of histomoniasis. NOT CLEARED FOR GAMEBIRDS.

TOXICITY: Growth depression, drop in egg production, nervous signs, ataxia, incoordination, convulsions, and death. DEADLY TO GEESE, DUCKS, AND PIGEONS. Early signs are reversible. Nerve damage is irreversible.

DOSAGE: CHICKENS and TURKEYS: 0.01875% level in feed
About 3 g/gal in water.

NOTE: FOLLOW DOSAGE DIRECTIONS ON THE PRODUCT LABEL WHEN USING THIS PRODUCT WITH WATER.

QUINIDINE OR ATABRINE (Overdose) (Human Drugs)

ACTIVITY: Treatment for malaria, Plasmodium, Haemaproteus, and Leucocytozoonosis.

TOXICITY: Acute death, nervousness, anorexia, severity of signs are in proportion to dosage intake, hot weather, and inadequate water supply.

DOSAGE: Calculate on basis of actual body mass (i.e., weight) of birds treated or (mg/lb body mass basis) as if product is to be administered to mammals.

ANTIBIOTICS (OVERDOSE)

Antibiotics are naturally occurring substances secreted by strepto-myces fungal organisms. The substances are toxic to pathogenic bac-teria that cause illness in gamebirds and other animals.

Most antibiotics are limited in their spectrum of activity, and therefore are prescribed as treatment against specific diseases. Antibiotics are considered bacteriocidal or bacteriostatic. Bacteriocidal medicines kill the invading pathogen on contact but the bacteriostatic drug stops or controls the growth and reproduction of the pathogen until it dies.

The rule of antibiotic therapy is do not use bacteriocidal and bacterio-static drugs similtaneously; however, it was shown recently that com-bination therapy can be beneficial in specific situations.

ANTIBIOTIC ACTIONS

BACTERIOCIDAL:	FDA APPROVED	ACTION AGAINST
Pencillin-G	Yes	G +, MG
Cephalosporins	No	G -
Aminoglycosides (Neomycin)	Yes	G -
Trimethoprim/Sulfa (Rofenaid)	Yes	G -,Coxy
Nitrofuran (NFZ)	Yes	G -
Nitroimidazole (Emtryl)	R_x only	Histomona
Quinolones (Baytril)	R_x only	G -, MG
Benzimidazole (TBZ)	Yes	Worms, Histo
BACTERIOSTATIC:		
Tetracyclines	Yes	G -
Chloramphenicol	No	G +/-
Macrolides (Tylan, Erythro)	Yes	G -/+,MG
Lincosamides	Yes	G +/-, MG
Novobiocin	Yes	G +
Spectinomycin	Yes	G +
Sulfas (SDM, SQ)	Yes	G +/-
Bacitracin	Yes	G +/-

The following listing enmumerates the specific ANTIBIOTIC; the diseases or syndromes with which it is effective, i.e., ACTIVITY; side effects if the drug is improperly used, TOXICITY; and DOSAGE,the amount and method of administration.

AMINOGLYCOSIDES

STREPTOMYCIN

ACTIVITY: Gram negative aerobic bacteria and certain gram positive anaerobic bacterins. Used with Penicillin as a broad-sprectrum antibiotic.

TOXICITY: Ototoxicity (hearing loss), neuroblock, renal damage

DOSAGE: CHICKENS — 75 g/ton in feed

                TURKEYS — 100 g/ton in feed

                        Pen-Strep @ 180 g/ton in feed

                CHICKENS — 1 to 1.5 tsp/gal (25% solution)

                        = 10 to 15 mg/lb body weight

                        Use for 3 to 5 days in water

NEOMYCIN

ACTIVITY: Clostridium and Coliforms, used with oxytetracycline (Neo-terra)

TOXICITY: Drug resistance by bacteria

DOSAGE: ALL SPECIES — 140 g/ton in feed

                    200 mg/gal in water

GENTAMICIN

ACTIVITY: Broad-spectrum gram positive and gram negative bacteria at present cleared only for injection in turkeys at 1 day of age. NOT FDA-CLEARED FOR GAME BIRDS

TOXICITY: Renal damage, aplastic anemia, death

DOSAGE: NOT FDA-CLEARED FOR GAME BIRDS

PENICILLIN

PENICILLIN
(G, V, AMPI, AMOXICILLIN)

ACTIVITY: Gram positive bacteria, staphylococcus, streptococcus, and clostridium (Quail Disease)

(CONTINUES)

PENICILLIN (CONTINUED)

TOXICITY: Anaphylactic shock, skin reaction, fever, and heart failure. DO NOT USE PROCAINE PENICILLIN ON: GUINEA PIGS, CHINCHILLA, BIRDS, SNAKES, or TURTLES. These animals are sensitive to the procaine radical.

DOSAGE: QUAIL: 20 g/ton in feed

PHEASANT: 50 g/ton in feed

CAUTION: 100g/ton MAXIMUM

EITHER SPECIES: 100,000 IU or 100 mg/gal in water

10,000 to 30,000 IU/kg or
1 to 3 mg/2.2 lb body weight by injection.

QUINOLONES

BAYTRIL
(ENROFLOXACIN)

Currently not cleared for gamebirds and poultry. Other quinolones are being developed.

ACTIVITY: *E. coli*, Salmonella, Pasteurella, Mycoplasma

TOXICITY: Vomiting, diarrhea, skin rash, photosensitivity

DOSAGE: Used in low doses in feed or water. Product trials for use in poultry are currently in progress.

100,000 IU or 100 mg/gal in water.

TETRACYCLINE

AUREOMYCIN, TERRAMYCIN, TETRACYCLINE [Three forms of this anitibiotic]:

ACTIVITY: Broad-spectrum - especially gram negative bacteria (Coliform, Pasteurella, Salmonella)

TOXICITY: Chelates calcium, contributing to rickets in young birds, enhances growth of yeasts and molds, and may cause a drug-resistance in bacteria.

DOSAGE: 100 to 200 g/ton in feed

200 to 800 mg/gal in water

PESTICIDES

Pesticides are chemical and other substances used to control external parasites on animals and plants. There are several types of pesticides, including those derived from certain plant tissues (rotenone, pyrethrum, and nicotine), chemical compounds of chlorinated hydrocarbon origin (organochlorine), and organophosphorous (OP) compounds. Organochlorines have been curtailed in use because of tissue residues and chronic toxicity. OP pesticides have now essentially replaced the organochlorines.

Only plant-derived and OP pesticides are FDA-approved for use on gamebirds and poultry. Only the OP compounds will be addressed here. The activity and toxicity of the approved organophosphates for avian species are similar; they are, therefore, discussed generically.

Pesticides:
ORGANOPHOSPHATES (Also See External Parasites)

ACTIVITY: Control of external lice and mites on birds. The OP is applied as dust or spray to birds (for lice and northern fowl mite) or environment. Several different pesticides are cleared for use on gamebirds and poultry. OP applied in this manner is rapidly inactivated in the body.

TOXICITY: If applied as granules or dust on litter and then eaten by the bird, OP pesticides are lethal. Rapid death occurs with a toxic dose or exposure. Toxic action is by cholinesterase reactivators. Diagnosis is based on finding OP activity in the crop and gizzard contents and in the muscle tissue.

DOSAGE: Follow instructions on product label for dilution and application. Always wear protective clothing and breathing apparatus to avoid extensive skin exposure and OP inhalation.

RODENTICIDES

Many poisons have been used against rodent pests. Farm animals, pets, gamebirds, and wildlife often gain access to these poisons, either through the baits or by eating poisoned dead rodents. Rodenticides must be used with caution. A pest-control specialist should be consulted before any major rodent control program is initiated.

Rodenticides:

ANTU, ARSENICALS, COMPOUND 1080, STRYCHNINE, WARFARIN, PHOSPHORUS, and ZINC PHOSPHIDE

ACTIVITY: For control of mice and rats in and around gamebird pens. The rodenticide must be available to the rodent but not to the gamebirds, pets, or wildlife. Special 'bait boxes' are available; these are built so as to permit the rodent to get to the poison, but birds and other animals can not.

TOXICITY: Depression, anorexia, prostration, and death. Lesions are pulmonary edema, swollen liver, muscle degeneration, hydropericardium, unclotted blood in trachea, respiratory failure (strychnine), hemorrhage (warfarin), opisthotonos, enteritis, ataxia, and convulsion (Zn phosphide).

DOSAGE: Use according to label instruction. Be alert to signs of toxicity in pets and other animals whenever rodenticides are used. Keep dead rodents picked up and buried or burned. Never feed dead rodents to other animals – birds, pets, or swine.

HEAVY METALS

In earlier times, metals were used in manufacturing a variety of products, e.g., antiseptics, paints, pesticides, and industrial compounds. Today, less-toxic materials have been substituted for many toxic metals.

Only lead and mercury will be discussed here. Lead was previously used in pesticides and still is used in all wet-cell batteries. Mercury is a component of industrial wastes that pollutes lakes in the area where such waste is dumped. In bird and animal poisonings, heavy metals concentrate in the liver and kidney tissues, as this is the location where the metals are detoxified and eliminated by the body. Poisoning occurs from accidental events such as feeding treated seed or exposure to water from industrial wastes. Always submit suspected cases to the Diagnostic Laboratory for confirmation.

Heavy Metals:

MERCURY (Hg)

ACTIVITY: Fungicides, topical ointments, antifungal seed-treatments, and industrial uses. (Most environmental mercury pollution is from industrial waste discharged into lakes and waterways.)

TOXICITY: Nonspecific but progressive impairment, with clinical signs of anorexia, enteritis, and nephritis (kidney damage). Lethal dose shows paralysis and neurological signs before death.

DOSAGE: Not used in medicines for gamebirds and poultry. Confirm suspicions of Hg toxicity with diagnosis from Poultry Diagnostic Laboratory.

LEAD (Pb)

ACTIVITY: Components of paints and clay soils. Used in fishing equipment and dry-cell batteries. Also found in dust around smelters and other lead-beneficiation plants. Generally widespread in the environment.

TOXICITY: Ingestion of lead progresses into lead poisoning. Wild waterfowl are at great risk from eating lead shot. Clinical signs of chronic illnesses are weight loss, ataxia, anorexia, weakness, prostration, anemia, green diarrhea, and death.

(CONTINUES)

DOSAGE: Not used in medicines. Confirm suspicion of poison with diagnosis from a Poultry Diagnostic Laboratory.

ALGAE

Several species of blue-green algae on warm fresh water lakes and ponds produce toxic substances that may poison birds and livestock that ingest the algae.

ACTIVITY: No beneficial activity. Algae are not used intentionally in gamebird, poultry, or livestock production. Poisonings are seasonal in Summer and Fall when algae bloom forms on water impoundments. Blooms concentrate on the down-wind side of the lake. Such areas should be 'fenced off' to prevent animals from drinking the water.

TOXICITY: Toxicity varies with algae's concentration. Signs from acute death (within minutes) to nervousness, paralysis, death (ducks), cyanosis, congested heart, swollen liver, and hepatocell necrosis. Diagnosis is confirmed by the identification of the toxin in the water.

DOSAGE: Not used intentionally. Algae poisonings are accidental events.

GROWER'S REFERENCE

ON

GAMEBIRD HEALTH

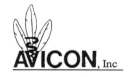

AVICON, Inc

BEHAVIOR

In birds and animals, much of the 'standard' (i.e., organized) behavior is recognized to be a part of the genetic programming of the species. Inherent reactive, ingestive, and kinetic actions represent the major behavioral activity that includes reaction, interaction, ingestion, grooming, exploration, territorialism, and rest.

Behavioral homeostasis, as much as physique, determines the animal's biological fitness and, in turn, its ability to compete and survive in the environment. Thus, a specie's typical behavior contributes to the animals biological fitness. Behavior is a continuum of components. Spatial and social behavioral activities are ethnological needs in the animal's function and adaptation to the environment and domestication. Behavior serves a number of purposes. Reactions are used for evading danger, expression, hierarchical status, and within-flock communication.

REACTIVE BEHAVIORS are the activities used by animals to live in harmony with their environment and to adjust to ecological changes. This is a learned behavior from association with penmates. Because of restricted opportunity for social activities, confined gamebirds may not be able to express typical highly organized behavior.

Specialized behaviors include:

REFLEX BEHAVIOR: Postural motions in response to pain.

GENERAL SOCIAL BEHAVIOR: The chick shows early response while still in the shell; for example, low pitch distress calls are emitted if eggs are cooled or rapid twittering if warmed. Newly hatched chicks are attracted to the hen by warmth, contact, clucking, and body movements. This attraction is greatest on the day of hatching. Chicks learn from the hen to eat, drink, roost, and avoid enemies. The attachment to the hen depends on the sound of her voice and her appearance.

As the down disappears from the head of the babies, the hen rejects the chicks. She pecks at them and the clutch starts to disperse and becomes more independent. The clutch or brood is the basic flock organization. Birds raised singly do not do as well in social adjustments as birds reared in a group.

Flock formation of adult birds relies on mutual tolerance and acceptance. Strange birds are first attacked, then slowly allowed to integrate into the flock but at the bottom of the social order.

SOCIAL BEHAVIOR OF TURKEYS: Domestic and wild turkeys have similar flocking patterns and social organization. The social dominance order is less stable than with chickens. Certain varieties of turkeys are dominant over other turkeys. For example, the black turkey is dominant over the bronze; the bronze is dominant over the gray, etc. In mixed sex groupings, the male is dominant over the female. Poults move about freely shortly after hatching and become imprinted to the hen during the first 1 to 2 days. Poults form groups and cluster together for warmth and feed. They wander as groups. Adult wild turkeys form large flocks for association and feeding during the winter. The flock breaks up at the onset of the breeding season but will regroup in fall until the next breeding season.

SOCIAL BEHAVIOR OF DUCKS: Wild mallards are monogamous and stay together from midwinter until nesting and incubation, a period of 5 months. In confinement production, this may not be possible if sex numbers are not balanced. Males display singly or in groups toward particular females. The display of females alternates from threatening to submissive gestures with a peculiar call. The submission is toward the preferred male, who then swims ahead of the hen but turns his nape toward her.

Paired birds leave the flock. The drake protects the hen during the time she is laying eggs. Incubation is 28 days. Hatchlings leave the nest the first day. The hen undergoes her annual molt during the 6- to 8-week brooding period before the hatchlings can fly.

Muscovy males are twice as heavy as the female and are aggressive toward other males. The male display is primitive and calls are simple. When startled, the hen emits a weak or feeble quack and the drake hisses, raises the crest, and shakes his tail. Swinging the head is a threat to other drakes and a courtship ritual to hens. After mating, the hen retires to her nest. The nest is not continuously occupied until incubation begins with the last one or two eggs of the clutch. The eggs hatch in 35 days. The drake sexually attacks any hen and does not participate in nesting, incubation, or care for the young.

OTHER BEHAVIOR RESPONSES: Avoidance and submission, agonistic, ingestion, body care, motion, exploratory, territorial, rest, and sleep.

CANNIBALISM

Cannibalism is the pecking, until death, of birds by their penmates. This is a behavioral problem that often develops into a vice. A vice is defined as a serious fault of character, evil conduct, depravity, fault, defect or blemish.

Cannibalism often begins as feather picking while the birds are only a few weeks old, and becomes a pattern of behavior that usually continues within the flock even though all known causative environmental, nutritional, and husbandry conditions may have been corrected. Poultry scientists have learned that any one or combination of stressors serve as the trigger that leads to serious feather picking and cannibalism. These include crowding, high light intensities, poor ventilation, high room temperature, high humidity, and low salt. Other triggering events are trace-nutrient deficiencies, insufficient feeding and drinking space, nervous and excitable birds (hereditary), external parasites, presence of sick or injured birds, boredom or idleness, and stress during transport.

The "peck order," not to be confused with cannibalism, is a function used by birds to establish a social order within the flock. The phenomenon is typical of all terrestrial-type birds, especially those maintained in larger flocks or in confined rearing and maintenance programs.

CONTROLLING CANNIBALISM:

Several species of poultry and gamebirds are notorious for cannibalism; therefore, control of cannibalism should be part of every grower's regular production procedure. When addressing the problem, review the list of causes known to be contributive to pecking, and correct any that are present. In young birds, crowding (within the pen or at the feeder and water fountain) is often the problem. Provide enough feeder space so that all birds can feed at the same time.

If pecking continues after all stressor conditions are corrected, other procedures may be required to stop cannibalism. Beak trimming, wearing specks or blinders, establishing good ground covers in outdoor pens, correcting the diet, and darkening the room may be helpful. Having plenty of feeder and drinking fountain space is a first requirement.

There are different forms of cannibalism and pecking —

TERRITORY - Breeder males will fight (peck) for territory.

VENT PECKING - Birds pecking at their own vent regions or the vent regions of others, and /or being pecked by penmates is sometimes caused by enteric infections in baby birds, by infections that affect the bursa of Fabricius, or by hens laying large eggs.

FEATHER PULLING is frequently seen in birds closely confined, especially if young flocks are crowded during brooding periods.

TOE PECKING is common in baby to juvenile birds and is initiated by hunger. Toe pecking is also a problem in certain specialty birds (e.g., hackle strains, jungle fowl, and gamefowl).

HEAD PECKING follows injuries to the head and fleshy portions of the face.

NOSE PECKING is an unusual form of cannibalism seen in 2- to 7-week old quail. It is so named because penmates peck at the fleshy (cere) portion of upper beak.

PROCEDURES TO PREVENT CANNIBALISM:

BEAK NOTCHING is used in day-old pheasant. A notch is burned into the upper beak, stopping the growth of the beak in front of the notch. Chicks have time to learn to eat and drink normally as it takes 10 to 14 days for the tip of the beak to fall off. As the beak grows out, it may have to be trimmed again.

BEAK TRIMMING, is the process of removing a portion of the beak, used on birds older than one day. The upper beak is shortened, rendering the bird ineffective at pecking. Beak trimming is a radical procedure, performed with an electrically heated blade, providing simultaneous cutting and cauterization. Severe trims create permanent damage. Before using this procedure, it is wise to consult an experienced producer or service company on age and standards of beak trimming. Try other methods of stopping cannibalism first.

STOPPING CANNIBALISM:

PROTECT, by isolation, the bird victims.

REMOVE offending birds.

PROVIDE ESCAPE AREAS — hiding areas indoor and ground cover outdoors.

SPECKS (BLINDERS) — These look like opaque spectacles for birds. They fit over the upper beaks and are held in place with a plastic pin through nostrils. Birds retain peripheral vision but cannot see dead ahead.

CROOKED NECK

Crooked-neck in birds is normally the resultant of one or a combination of causes — injury, heredity, and infection, producing muscle spasms in the neck or structural damage to the cervical vertebrae. Crooked necks in gamebirds are the result of a neck injury suffered from having flown into a wall, window pane, or other solid object.

In poultry, however, a "crooked neck" malady is probably caused by a genetic predisposition. A study by Morehead and Mohammed reported on a flock of turkeys in which 10 percent of the birds were affected. The principal lesion was osteodystrophy (deformity of neck vertebrae).

The clinical signs were similar to those of a crooked-neck syndrome attributed to a single recessive hereditary gene. The workers concluded that osteodystrophy of the neck was not hereditary, but infectious, in nature. The author has seen turkey flocks with high incidences of crooked neck in which the cause was staphylococcal septicemia. The condition occurred in male birds that at puberty had spent considerable time strutting. The flock responded to medication with penicillin. Crooked-neck must be controlled on an individual flock basis. Birds with crooked-neck should not be saved as breeder replacements for the following year.

FOWL HYSTERIA

Fowl hysteria, sometimes called hyperexcitability or alarm reaction, is a syndrome affecting semimature and mature birds. The condition is characterized by extreme nervousness, flightiness, and intermittent but regular stampeding. Flocks with hysteria develop a regular pattern of stampeding that recurs without apparent stimuli.

The cause, behavioral in nature (there is no evidence of an infectious agent), is believed to be brought on by crowding. Contributing factors may complicate the situation. Factors that may contribute to the onset or seriousness of the condition include:

MALNUTRITION - West Coast poultry health workers equate hysteria in pullets with a protein deficiency.

VITAMIN DEFICIENCY - Hysteria in some flocks has been alleviated by adding extra niacin to the ration. Niacin and thiamin (members of the B vitamin family) play a role in the health of the nervous system, and niacin is a component of enzymes involved in digestion.

HEREDITARY FACTORS - Workers at Ohio State University with nine flocks in 1962 concluded that hysteria is a recessive inheritance trait.

TRAUMA - A 1969 Washington State University report concluded that pain from toenail wounds produced hysteria in highly nervous flocks. Removing toenails with a beak-trim machine reduced the incidence of hysteria.

STRAY VOLTAGE — Electrical currents exceeding 0.5 volt will stimulate hysteria. In 1993, stray electrical voltage was the cause of hysteria in mature leghorn hens. In most cases, the voltage enters the house through the water system; however, finding the source of the stray voltage is necessary to correct the problem.

CLINICAL SIGNS:

Flightiness and, hyperexcitability in juvenile or mature birds are the primary clinical signs. Hysteria flocks exhibit signs of panic by running, flying, and squawking as if attacked by a predator.

PATHOLOGY:

Gross signs are various stages of molt with an absence of serious external lesions in birds of the same age. A typical flock history is progressive flightiness and increased frequency of panic seizures. Affected birds lose weight and decrease production. Pathogenic organisms are absent.

CONTROL:

Make certain the problem is hysteria.

Move birds to new surroundings, e.g., another pen or facility with different equipment.

Assure a comfortable environment. Light intensity, temperature, humidity, and ventilation should not stress the birds.

Increase protein level in feed by 1 or 2 percent.

Niacin therapy [200 g/ton] in feed for 5 to 7 days and vitamins and electrolytes containing thiamin in the drinking water for 3 to 6 days.

Check premises and equipment for stray electrical voltage. Have power company ground all sources subject to stray voltage

Provide biosecurity and good husbandry to assure comfort, nutrition, and nonstressful environment for current and successive flocks. Eliminate the factors known to cause hysteria.

Select docile breeds.

QUAIL HYSTERIA: John Mullin describes quail hysteria as "fast-forward hysteria" that is a behavioral trait in all quail. Quail dart "fast-forward" every time they become alarmed. As a result, their running into open unprotected areas will get them into trouble. Control is directed at brooding and environment. Eliminate corners in hover to prevent piling and smothering. Try to discourage running. Nonrunning birds will be better at "holding and flushing" when mature, providing a better challenge to the gun dog and the hunter.

GRAY PARTRIDGE: The gray partridge retains a high level of wildness in captivity. Cannibalism and hysteria can be serious problems. Partridge hysteria apparently differs from fowl hysteria, as it seems to begin with gang cannibalism attacks on a single bird. The assaulted bird's terrified calls 'trigger' panic and frenzy in all the birds in the pen. From that point, the condition fits the pattern of fowl hysteria. In partridge, hysteria is prevalent in 6- to 7-week-old birds with reoccurrence at 11 to 15 weeks of age.

PENDULOUS CROP

Pendulous crops, also referred to as sour crop, crop impaction, and crop binding, occur in immature birds. The crop becomes distended with sour-smelling contents that are usually semi-liquid but may include dry undigested feed or litter. Work in Florida shows that baby birds brooded on sand may ingest such large quantities of sand that the crop becomes static. The sand is so heavy that intestinal peristalsis is unable to move the sand through the digestive tract. Seriously affected birds die.

Pendulous crop in domestic poultry occurs in low incidence in chickens and turkeys and even less in gamebirds. It is a hereditary predisposition, although depraved eating habits can cause the bird to habitually eat sand or litter, mechanically inducing a pendulous crop condition. On a hot day, individual birds will consume so much water that its weight causes a pendulous crop. Birds continue to eat but digestion is impaired. The condition can be surgically corrected on individual birds of high value.

Birds with pendulous crop should be eliminated from the flock and never saved for breeder replacements. Normal incidence in commercial poultry ranges from 1 to 5 percent. Culling and disposing the few affected birds within the flock is the most economical method of control.

PICKING

Birds use their beaks in eating, self-defense, and attack. They can be vicious in attacking pen mates. Usually such harmful activity — feather picking, head picking, nose picking (in quail), and toe picking — can be prevented if the flock manager is aware of contributive factors and promptly alleviates unfavorable conditions.

FEATHER PICKING: Dull and broken feathers with bare-skin patches on the neck, back, tail, and vent areas provide evidence of feather picking. Tail picking is common in growing birds before new feathers, filled with blood, become dense enough to cover the skin. Crowded conditions, lack of exercise, external parasites, and low dietary protein or other nutrients are contributing causes for feather picking.

Birds of all ages and species, including pheasants, quail, partridge, ducks, turkeys, and chickens can be feather pickers. Loss of feathers may be through the natural process of molting or a result of mating activities. during the breeding season. Many immature flocks, however, do experience aggressive feather picking.

The most common method for controlling feather picking is trimming the beak, thus rendering the birds incapable of pecking or picking. [Beak trimming is discussed in the presentation on "Cannibalism," page 333.] Feed should be evaluated because feed low in protein will cause the birds to crave feathers — either picked or molted. Light-intensity control, isolation and protection of victims of feather pickers, supplementation of the ration, increased space per bird, and trimmed beaks are all husbandry procedures employed to prevent or control feather picking. Prevention is important because feather picking leads to cannibalism, and cannibalism can cause the loss of many birds.

HEAD PICKING: Head picking often follows injuries to the head, especially in older birds. Birds that experience frost bite or are bleeding as a result of a fight become target birds for head picking. Head picking is most common in caged birds, occuring when birds in adjacent cages pick at head and face through the wire. Even when beaks have been trimmed, head picking still occurs; therefore, in caged birds it is recommended that visual barriers be installed between the cages.

NOSE PICKING IN QUAIL: In quail, nose picking is an unusual form of cannibalism. The birds attack their penmates by picking at the nose (cere) where the fleshy portion merges with the beak above the nares. Nose picking is more prevalent in 2- to 7-week-old birds in crowded pens. Victims that survive may have permanently damaged beaks;

some victims bleed to death.

Nose picking occurs only in artificial-brooding operations; it does not occur in the wild. Like a bad habit, this vice is extremely difficult to eliminate once it gets started in a pen. Quail growers should be alert to nose picking during early brooding. To curb the problem, try a variety of management changes similar to those suggested in feather picking. One observer found that adding meat by-products to the feed ration was helpful in the prevention and control of nose picking.

TOE PICKING: Toe picking has been seen in gamebirds, ducks, and some chicken flocks. The cause is hunger, especially in birds reared on paper to prevent the birds from eating litter. To prevent toe picking, use feeder lids or sprinkle feed on paper under and around the brooder.

Toe picking also occurs when wire-brooded quail and chukar cuts a toe or foot; sight of these injuries seem to trigger onset of the syndrome. If toe-picking begins and birds are injured, use red bulbs under brooder. In this light, chicks do not easily detect blood or scabs on feet and toes of penmates.

Toe picking is also a problem in breeding flocks of specialty strains of birds, especially in gamefowl and birds grown for hackle feathers. In "hackle" strains, the hens pick the toes of the roosters. Light control is helpful but does not fully stop or eliminate the problem.

VENT PICKING: Picking in the vent and abdominal regions is the most severe form of cannibalism, since it escalates rapidly and often results in the death of the victim. Vent picking is less prevalent in gamebirds or turkeys than in chickens. Young chickens infected with infectious bursal disease (IBD) will often pick their vent. IBD irritates the bursa of Fabricius, located just above the vent.

In older birds, vent picking is usually associated with egg production. Hens that lay large eggs may prolapse as the egg is laid. Then other birds in the pen or cage attack this hen. This condition is also called "prolapse" and "pick-out."

SMOTHERING

Smothering is generally caused by birds piling in a corner or over-crowding. Certain species of gamebirds are more prone than others to piling. Every producer of gamebirds is conscious of the potential problem and watches for birds piling and smothering. In the majority of the cases, an incident (loud noise, lightning flash, fright) causes panic that results in the birds piling and dying. Death is from suffocation. Chilled and sick young birds seeking warmth are prone to piling.

Storms, power outages, loss of heat, and bird discomfort during thunderstorms will cause panic, leading to piling and death. In hot weather, live birds transported in tight containers or closed car trunks may smother to death. Sick birds have a lower resistance to environmental stress; therefore smothering may be greater in sick or convalescent flocks.

Gamebird and poultry producers have learned that the use of a chick guard around the brooder stove can prevent great losses from piling and smothering. Young birds and flocks moved into different quarters need to be checked frequently until the flock has adapted to the new pens and equipment. Control relies on a quick diagnosis to correct the cause, including medication when an infection is the source.

WINDPUFF

Windpuff is thought to be the result a rupture of an airsac with the escaped air trapped under the skin of the neck and upper body. Windpuff is also called emphysema, but emphysema is an incorrect term. True emphysema is a breakdown of the interior structure of the lungs.

With windpuffs, the lungs fill with air but the affected bird is unable to exhale or release the air. The individual becomes barrel-chested. However, the air is under the skin and can be released by inserting a sterile hypodermic needle into the air pocket. Affected birds may have to have the air released twice or more. Most recover without medication or further incident.

Windpuff occurs in birds from 1 to 21 days of age, but in juvenile and adult birds windpuff often leads to infection in the subcutaneous region of the trapped air. This condition is called cellulitis. Cellulitis is an infectious process that does not respond to medication. Such birds have a mushy-foamy texture to the touch. The condition may affect only one side of the body of the bird. Even though cellulitis is not contagious, when this condition is discovered, the economically prudent decision is to promptly cull and humanely dispose of all affected birds. Cellulitis birds are not useful for release and require considerable trimming if slaughtered.

GLOSSARY

Definitions of some technical terms used frequently in this manual.

ABSORPTION:
Take up of fluids or substances.

ACQUIRED IMMUNITY:
Immunity achieved by recovery from disease or response to vaccine.

ADHERE:
To stick or cling to something.

ADSORPTION:
Attachment of a substance to the surface of another.

AEROBIC:
With oxygen. Aerobic microorganisms require oxygen for growth.

AGENT:
Organism or substance capable of causing illness or disease.

AGGLUTINATION:
Clumping of cells in a fluid.

AGGLUTINATION TITER:
Highest dilution of a serum that causes clumping of antigen.

AIRSACCULITIS:
Inflammation of the air sacs.

ANAEROBIC:
Microorganisms that do not require oxygen to reproduce and grow.

ANEMIA:
Loss of RBC. Below normal blood count for animal species, age, and sex.

ANTIBODY:
Natural or vaccine-induced globulin that counteracts toxins or pathogens.

ANTIGEN:
A substance that causes production of antibodies.

ANTISERUM:
Serum from immune animal(s).

APHIS:
Animal and Plant Health Inspection Service. The USDA agency that oversees.animal health, import and export.

ARBOVIRUS:
Arthropod-borne viri that causes encephalitis, etc.

ARTICULAR:
Relating to the joint.

ASPHYXIATION:
Blockage of the trachea. Suffication.

ASSIMILATION:
The conversion of absorbed food into the substance of the body.

AUTOGENOUS VACCINE:
Vaccine manufactured from bacteria cultured from birds in the infected flock.

BACKYARD FLOCK:
A noncommercial poultry enterprise.

BACTERIA:
A class of microbes larger than viruses.

BACTERIN:
Bacterial vaccine.

BIOSECURITY:
Measures to prevent introduction of disease to flock or premises.

BIOTIN:
Colorless, crystalline B vitamin.

BREEDERS:
Birds selected specifically to produce eggs for hatching.

BROODER:
Warm, draft-free housing for baby chicks.

BURSA OF FABRICIUS:
A lymphoid organ above the cloaca in young birds.

CALCIFICATION:
Hardening of tissues because of calcium inclusion.

CASEOUS:
Resembling cheese or curds; cheesy.

CATARRH:
Inflammation of the mucous membrane with a free discharge of exudate.

CECUM:
Blind pouch.Poultry have two ceca, attached to intestine at the iliocecal junction.

CELLULITIS:
Inflammation of subcutaneous tissue.

CHOLINE:
Vitamin-like chemical substance vital to liver functions.

CLINICAL SIGNS:
Typical signs of a disease. Symptons.

CLOACA:
Cavity common to reproductive, digestive, and urinary systems.

CLUMPING:
See *Agglutination*.

COCCIDIOSTAT
Medicinal agent mixed in feed or drinking water to control coccidiosis.

CONDYLES:
Articular prominence of a bone.

CORN- SOYBEAN RATION:
Feed consisting of corn & soybean meal. Cereal grains may be used.

CORONAVIRUS:
Major group of animal viruses.

CROP:
Dilatation of esophagus of birds where food is stored.

CULTURE:
Propagation of microorganism or living tissue cells in special laboratory media.

CYANOSIS:
Bluish discoloration of tissues due to lack of oxygen in the blood.

CYANOTIC:
Bluish in color, indicating cyanosis.

DEFICIENCY:
A lack of essential nutrients such as vitamins, minerals, or amino acids.

DIETARY ROLE:
Activity pertaining especially to the diet, digestion, and or assimilation.

DOSE:
Quantity of medication to be given at one time.

EMBRYONIC DEATH:
Death of the chick in the egg.

ENDEMIC:
Recurrence of disease outbreak within a flock or area.

ENDOCARDITIS:
Inflammation of the endocardium.

ENDOCARDIUM
Tissue lining the heart and valves.

ENTERITIS:
Inflammation of intestine.

ENZYME:
Secretion by living cells that aid metabolism.

EPIDEMIC:
An acute, explosive outbreak in an area or flock.

ERYTHROCYTES:
Red blood cells.

ESOPHAGUS:
Throat

EXPECTORATED:
Spit up.

FERAL BIRDS:
Wild birds.

FERTILITY:
Percent of fertile eggs.

FOCAL NECROSIS:
Local areas of dead tissue.

FOMITE:
Inanimate carrier of diseases.

FUNGUS:
Mold, yeast, smut, mushrooms, etc.

GIZZARD:
Muscular organ of the alimentary canal for grinding food.

GRAM-NEGATIVE:
Bacteria that stain pink from gram stain procedure.

GRAM-POSITIVE:
Bacteria that stain blue.

HATCHABILITY:
The number of eggs in a fertile set that hatch.

HEMADSORPTION:
Adherence of red blood cells to other cells.

HEMAGGLUTINATION:
Clumping of RBC due to, viruses, or chemical substances.

HEMATOCRIT:
Percentage of RBC in the blood.

HEMORRHAGE:
Loss of blood from the blood vessels; bleeding.

HISTOLOGY:
Microscopic study of tissues.

HISTOPATHOLOGICAL:
Microscopic lesions in diseased tissues.

HOST:
Animal or plant that harbors a parasite or pathogen.

HOST-SPECIFIC:
Single-host species.

ICOSOHEDRAL:
Polyhedron with twenty faces used to describe viruses.

IMMUNE:
Ability to resist infection from a normal exposure to a specific pathogen.

IMMUNIZATION:
Response to vaccination.

INACTIVATED VACCINE:
Vaccine of killed virus or bacteria.

INCLUSION BODIES:
Intracellular bodies thought to be viral particles.

INCUBATION:
Hatching chicks artificially.

INCUBATION PERIOD:
Time between exposure to a pathogen and onset of clinical signs.

INCUBATION TIME:
Time for eggs to hatch.

INCUBATOR:
Equipment used for hatching eggs.

INDUCED IMMUNITY:
Antibodies stimulated by vaccine.

INFECTION:
Presence of active pathogens in blood and/or tissues.

INFESTED:
Presence of parasitic organisms on the skin.

INGESTED:
Swallowed. Eaten.

INHERITED IMMUNITY:
Natural resistance to a disease.

INTERMEDIATE HOST:
Animal in which a parasite must spend part of its life cycle.

INTRANASAL:
In the nose.

INTRAOCULAR:
In the eye.

LARVAL STAGE:
Immature stages of some insects.

LENTOGENIC:
Low in virulence.

LESION:
Change in structure, color, or size of an organ or other part of the body.

LEUKOCYTES:
White blood cells (WBC).

LUMEN:
Channel or cavity in a tubular organ.

LYMPHOID:
Pertaining to the lymphatic cells, tissues, and system.

MACROSCOPIC:
Visible without magnification.

MALADY:
Disease or disorder of the birds.

MANGANESE:
A mineral, essential in animal diets. Symbol: Mn.

MESENTERY:
Thin membrane connecting intestines and the body wall; provides support for nerves and vessels.

MESOGENIC:
A medium virulence-pathogenicity.

METABOLISM:
Chemical and physical processes involved in growth.

MICROHEMATOCRAT:
Rapid test to measure packed RBC volume using tiny amounts of blood with a capillary tube and high-speed centrifuge.

MOLT:
Loss and replacement of feathers.

MORBID:
Sick. Ill.

MORBIDITY:
Relative incidence of a disease.

MUCOUS:
Secreting mucus; resembling mucus.

MUCUS:
Slime secreted by the mucous membranes.

MYCOPLASMA:
Any of the mycoplasma organisms.

MYCOSIS:
Any disease caused by a fungus.

MYOCARDIUM:
Heart muscle.

MYXOVIRUSES:
Viruses that hemagglutinate RBC.

NARES:
Nostrils.

NECROSIS:
Death and decomposition of tissue; focal or diffuse.

NECROTIC FOCI:
Focal necrosis.

NIACIN:
Nicotinic acid, a "B" vitamin.

ORNITHINE:
Birds with straight beaks.

ORTHOMYXOVIRUS:
Subgroup of myxoviruses. Primarily influenza.

PARENTAL IMMUNITY
Antibodies passed by hen to chick in the egg.

PARASITE:
An organism living at the expense of another animal host.

PASSERINE:
Free-flying song birds.

PASSIVE IMMUNITY:
Immunity from antibodies present in the egg.

PATHOGEN:
Disease agent.

PATHOGEN PRESSURE:
Level or number of infectious organisms within the area to which birds are exposed.

PATHOGENIC:
Capable of causing a disease.

PERICARDITIS:
Inflammation of the heart sac.

PERIHEPATITIS:
Inflammation of the liver capsule.

PERITONEUM:
Membrane lining the abdominal walls covering viscera.

PERITONITIS:
Inflammation of the peritoneum.

PEROSIS:
Leg deformity caused by deficiency of manganese (Mn).

PETECHIA:
Pinpoint hemorrhage.

PHALLUS:
Reproductive organ of the male bird.

PHARYNX:
Throat

PLASMA:
Fluid portion of blood that contains fibrin and serum.

PLEOMORPHIC:
Occurring in various forms.

PRIMARY HOST:
Animal in which parasite completes life cycle.

PROLIFERATIVE:
Growing by rapid reproduction of similar parts.

PROPORTIONER:
Device to meter medicine into drinking water.

PROTOZOA:
Microscopic one-celled organism.

PROVENTRICULUS:
Glandular stomach of the avian species.

PSITTACINE:
Birds with curved beaks; parrot family.

PUPAL:
Immature stage in life cycle of insects.

PURULENT:
Pus, exudate.

PUS:
Mixture of fluids, bacteria, and tissue cells. Exudates.

QUARANTINE:
To detain or isolate, by law, to stop spread of disease.

RBC:
Red blood cells

REOVIRUS:
Viruses of respiratory and enteric origin.

RESISTANT:
Possessing ability to avoid infection.

SALPINGITIS:
Inflammation of the oviduct or fallopian tubes of the hen.

SALVAGE FLOCKS:
Early slaughter of flocks after disease outbreak to minimize financial loss.

SENTINEL BIRDS:
Susceptible birds placed in a facility to detect latent infections.

SEPTICEMIA:
Infection of the blood by pathogenic microbes. Blood poison.

SEROLOGICAL TESTS or SEROLOGY:
Tests on serum for antibodies against specific diseases.

SEROSA:
Tissues supporting the organs.

SEROTYPE:
Classification of a microorganism based on cell wall antigens.

SERUM:
Fluid portion of blood remaining after clot is removed.

SYSTEMIC:
Throughout the body via the blood.

TITER:
Dilution of serum to neutralize a given quantity of antigen.

TOXIN:
Poisonous substance.

TOXOID:
Modified toxin to stimulate antibodies against the toxin.

TRACHEA:
Windpipe.

TRICHOMONADS:
Flagellated protozoan organism that infects digestive tract.

VACCINATION:
Inoculation with a vaccine to stimulate immunity.

VACCINE:
Antigens for use in vaccination.

VECTOR:
Arthropod that transmits disease.

VELOGENIC:
Highly virulent.

VIRULENT:
Highly pathogenic.

VIRUS:
Smallest disease-causing microbes.

VIRUS-LIKE:
Pathogenic organisms that act like viruses; susceptible to antibiotics.

VITAMINS:
Dietary substances essential in small amounts for normal metabolic functions in animals.

VITAMIN PREMIX:
Vitamin feed additive used for nutritional balance.

WATERFOWL:
Ducks, geese, and swans.
Swimmers.

WATER-DISPERSIBLE:
Soluble in water, for use in
drinking water.

WILD BIRDS:
See Feral Birds

INDEX

Dedicated pages appear in capital letters with bold numerals

SECTION INDEX